Connections Between
Spirit and Work in
Career Development

Connections Between Spirit and Work in Career Development

New Approaches and Practical Perspectives

Deborah P. Bloch and Lee J. Richmond, Editors

Davies-Black Publishing
Palo Alto, California

Published by Davies-Black Publishing, an imprint of Consulting Psychologists Press, Inc., 3803 East Bayshore Road, Palo Alto, CA 94303; 1-800-624-1765.

Special discounts on bulk quantities of Davies-Black books are available to corporations, professional associations, and other organizations. For details, contact the Director of Book Sales at Davies-Black Publishing, an imprint of Consulting Psychologists Press, Inc., 3803 East Bayshore Road, Palo Alto, CA 94303; 415-691-9123; Fax 415-988-0673.

Quotations on p. viii: From "What Work Is," by Philip Levine. Copyright © 1991 by Philip Levine. Reprinted by permission of Alfred A. Knopf, Inc.

Quotation on p. 56: From Vallas, S. P. "Comments and Observations." In *The Nature of Work,* K. Erikson and S. P. Vallas (Eds.). © 1990 Yale University Press. Reprinted with permission.

Quotation on pp. 258–259: From *The Prophet* by Kahlil Gibran. Copyright 1923 by Kahlil Gibran and renewed 1951 by Administrators C T A of Kahlil Gibran Estate and Mary G. Gibran. Reprinted by permission of Alfred A. Knopf, Inc.

01 00 99 98 97   10 9 8 7 6 5 4 3 2 1
Printed in the United States of America

Library of Congress Cataloging-in-Publication Data
Connections between spirit and work in career development : new approaches and
    practical perspectives / Deborah P. Bloch and Lee J. Richmond, editors.
        p. cm.
    Includes bibliographical references and index.
    ISBN 0-89106-105-3
    1. Career development.   2. Work—Psychological aspects.   I. Bloch, Deborah P.
    II. Richmond, Lee J.
HF5381.C686   1997
650.1—dc21
                                                                    97-15339
                                                                    CIP

FIRST EDITION
First printing 1997

Contents

Introduction

Deborah P. Bloch
University of San Francisco

In 1933, Jung's *Modern Man in Search of a Soul* was first published in English. In it, Jung describes what he calls "the general neurosis of our time." "About a third of my cases," he writes, "are suffering from no clinically definable neurosis, but from the senselessness and emptiness of their lives." He continues, "It is difficult to treat patients of this particular kind by rational methods, because they are in the main socially well-adapted individuals of considerable ability, to whom normalization means nothing. . . . The ordinary expression for this situation is: 'I am stuck'" (Jung, 1931/1933, p. 61).

In contrast, poet Donald Hall (1993) describes in *Life Work* his "best day." "The best day begins with waking early—I check the clock: damn! it's only 3:00 a.m.—because I want so much to get out of bed and start working. Usually something particular beckons so joyously—like a poem that I have good hope for, that seems to go well. Will it look as happy today as it looked yesterday?" Almost agonizing over the delay, he exquisitely paints his impatience to get out of bed, the coffee making, the details of the morning until he finishes breakfast reading the paper. And then, he writes,

> As I approach the end of the *Globe* saving the sports section until last, I feel work-excitement building, job-pressure mounting—until I need resist it no more but sit at the desk and open the folder that holds the day's beginning, its desire and its hope. Then I lose myself. In the best part of the best day, *absorbedness* occupies me from footsole to skulltop. (p. 41)

What is this sense of "absorbedness"? How do some people find it while others feel "stuck" in meaningless lives? The vivid contrast between feeling stuck and being absorbed by work is presented by Philip Levine (1991) in the title poem of the collection *What Work Is*. The narrator begins:

> We stand in the rain in a long line
> waiting at Ford Highland Park. For work.
> You know what work is—if you're
> old enough to read this you know what
> work is, although you may not do it.
> Forget you. This is about waiting,

Then, as he shifts from one foot to another, he thinks about his brother, at home sleeping after his "miserable night shift at Cadillac," work the brother does so that he may study German, to sing Wagner. Overcome by love, the narrator asks himself why he has never expressed his love to his brother:

> not because you're too young or too dumb,
> not because you're jealous or even mean
> or incapable of crying in
> the presence of another man, no
> just because you don't know what work is.
> (pp. 18–19)[1]

Work, in the beginning of the poem, is hard, unrewarding labor. Embittered, the worker challenges the reader. "Forget you," he says. This poem is about me, about my waiting, about my doing and waiting to do. We all know, he says, in this same tone, how dampening (like the rain) to the spirit work is. But then he thinks of his brother's devotion to an art and its craft, the learning of German, and suddenly recognizes another kind of work that he does not understand. This second kind of work is perhaps the kind that produces what Hall has called *absorbedness*.

Jung (1931/1933) suggests that the need to find meaning in life occurs somewhere around age forty, after the task of finding one's place in the work world. He suggests that this spiritual search is associated with a feminization of the man and briefly sketches the idea that women become more associated with manly traits in this same beginning middle age. It certainly remains unclear as to whether or not women and men experience the same set of tasks and challenges in their life-careers. However, many women writing about women have expressed the same longings for meaning in work to which Jung alludes for men.

Heilbrun (1988) has repeatedly written about the change in women's power and needs at this same middle period of the forties to fifties. "We must recognize what the past suggests: women are well beyond youth when they begin, often unconsciously, to create another story. Not even then do they recognize it as another story. Usually they believe that the obvious reasons for what they are doing are the only ones; only in hindsight, or through a biographer's imaginative eyes, can the concealed story be surmised" (pp. 109–110). Lindbergh (1955/1978) also writes about the growing pains of middle age in a woman's life: "One might be free for growth of mind, heart, and talent; free at last for spiritual growth; free of the clamping sunrise shell" (p. 88).

Indirectly, through the writers selected, this introduction begins to raise the questions of the book: First, how does one find meaning in work? The answers suggested in this initial exploration seem associated with what some might call spirituality, what others would identify as a sense of harmony between the internal and external realities, with a sense of preoccupation rather than occupation, with immersion in work. Second, questions of age have been raised. Do writers conclude that people seek meaning in their lives in their later years because that is when they, the writers, are coming to grips with this issue, or are there identifiable stages of career where meaning has different definitions? And there are gender-related questions: How is women's quest the same as or different from men's?

In this book, *Connections Between Spirit and Work in Career Development,* the chapter authors present their answers to the questions raised in this introduction and at the same time raise other questions salient to the overarching considerations of spirituality and work. All of the chapters are based upon strong theoretical bases and each draws conclusions that have implications for application, both by individuals and by the professionals helping them in their quest for meaning through career development. However, the chapters differ in their emphasis. The first six chapters lean more toward theory, whereas the remaining five have a stronger orientation toward application.

Each of the first six chapters explores the broad questions of the meaning of work through a different set of filters. In the first chapter, "The Spirit in Career Counseling: Fostering Self-Completion Through Work," Mark L. Savickas uses the filters of psychology and career development theory. He explores the relationships of spirit, character, and self-completion and describes the use of narrative in meaning making for the counselor and client. The second chapter, "Creating One's Personal Meaning Throughout the Cycles of Life: Its Development in Career, Psychosocial, and Faith Realms" by Beverly E. Eanes, continues the use of the theoretical filter of the behavioral sciences. She reviews and compares the life cycle stages of Erikson, the career development stages of Super, and the stages of faith developed by Fowler. The third chapter moves in a different direction. In "Work as Worth: Money or Meaning," Michael Demkovich turns to philosophy. He uses two lenses—the social-economic and the moral-ethical—to illuminate the answers to the questions of self, work, and society. David V. Tiedeman and Anna Miller-Tiedeman, in Chapters 4 and 5, draw upon systems theory and quantum mechanics as their theoretical filters. In "Ready, Set, Grow: An Allegoric Induction into Quantum Careering," Tiedeman engages in an imaginary conversation with Winnie-the-Pooh and friends to discuss the implications of the new scientific paradigms, particularly complexity and complementarity, for understanding human behavior. In "The Lifecareer® Process Theory: A Healthier Choice," Miller-Tiedeman describes the systems theory–based approach to understanding career and then links this understanding to wholeness and health. The final theoretical filter, that of Christian theology, is presented by Harvey L. Huntley, Jr., in the sixth chapter, "How Does 'God-Talk' Speak to the Workplace?: An Essay on the Theology of Work." After describing the traditional and contemporary theological approaches to meaning in the postmodern workplace, Huntley develops the idea of meaning as a dynamic experience that includes paid and unpaid work, leisure, and worship in balance both for individual spirituality and for the common good.

Part Two explores more specific applications to finding the connections between spirit and career. Marian Stoltz-Loike, in Chapter 7, deals with "Creating Personal and Spiritual Balance: Another Dimension in Career Development." After a concise review of the literature on work-family concerns, she presents a model for balancing life through work, relationships, and spiritual practice. In "Vocation as Calling: Affirmative Response or 'Wrong Number,'" Chapter 8, Carole A. Rayburn defines vocation broadly and then examines the barriers to following a vocation and the benefits of doing so. She stresses the transcendent nature of calling, first that it is not limited to any particular work and further that it is not limited by the sexual or racial stereotyping imposed by societal or institutional rules or roles. Chapter 9, by Deborah P. Bloch, "Spirituality, Intentionality, and Career Success: The Quest for Meaning," defines meaning as vocation or harmony and describes two ways of achieving it: the use of meditation, visualization, poetry, and other art forms; and the practice of intentionality (the movement of matter by the mind) to bring about changes. The latter includes a discussion of the relationship of intentionality to current work in subatomic physics. Lee J. Richmond, in Chapter 10, "Spirituality and Career Assessment: Metaphors and Measurement," discusses traditional career assessment instruments and instruments that are designed for spiritual assessment. In both cases, she examines the usefulness of the instruments in helping individuals find meaning in their work. The chapter stresses the uses of assessment instruments to connect the experiential, the intuitive, and the spiritual. In Chapter 11, "Inspiriting the Workplace: Developing a Values-Based Management System," Samuel M. Natale and Joanne C. Neher provide a series of steps that can be taken by organizations—at individual and corporate levels—to bring about a workplace based on values. They stress the need for a systems approach that incorporates affective, behavioral, and cognitive components to move the culture from one based on good as equated with purchasing power to one of spirituality. In the Epilogue, Lee J. Richmond tries to connect all the foregoing chapters.

As the authors presented their ideas about connections between spirit and work, many drew upon religious writings and experiences that held personal meaning for them. In reviewing the chapters, we noted that these writings and experiences drew most heavily from the Judeo-Christian tradition. In no way do we mean to suggest that connections between spirit and work are associated only with the religions mentioned or indeed with any religion. We appreciate the openness of the chapter authors and hope that all readers will be able to make the connections between spirit and work that are meaningful to them.

In any edited work, the order of the chapters is based on a mental model held by the editors. In planning and implementing this book, we saw a rationale for the order of chapters, a flow from one to the next. However, recurring themes among the chapters could very well have suggested other orders of presentation. Themes that arise in several or many of the chapters center on meaningfulness through the relationship of the self to others, through the relinquishing of self-absorption or egocentricity, through balance, through contributions to or identification with community, through change and process, and through prayer or stillness. All of the chapters deal with current issues and recognize the perils of the contemporary workplace with its volatile economics. Other connections among chapters occur in the wide range of literature cited, from the Bible and other sacred texts to psychology, philosophy, economics, and poetry to systems theory and quantum mechanics. The reader is encouraged to find the many links that exist among these separately authored works.

Finally, at the conclusion of the poem "Among School Children," William B. Yeats (1928/1962, p. 166) sings to us about the beauty of labor. He compares labor to dancing, cautioning us not to bruise our bodies for the sake of our souls, nor to seek "blear-eyed wisdom" by burning the proverbial "midnight oil." He speaks of the joy of harmony and wholeness in life and work; comparing the dancer to the chestnut tree in which the leaves, the flowers, and the root are all inseparable parts. And then he addresses the essence of connectedness as he asks the critical question: "O body swayed to music, O brightening glance, How can we know the dancer from the dance?" Let us hope that this book is offered and received not with "blear-eyed wisdom" but in the spirit of the dancer, each dancing a career to his or her personal melody of meaning.

REFERENCES

Hall, D. (1993). *Life work.* Boston: Beacon Press.

Heilbrun, C. G. (1988). *Writing a woman's life.* New York: Ballantine.

Jung, C. G. (1933). *Modern man in search of a soul.* (W. S. Dell & C. F. Baynes, Trans.). Orlando, FL: Harcourt Brace. (Original work published 1931)

Levine, P. (1991). *What work is.* New York: Knopf.

Lindbergh, A. M. (1978). *Gift from the sea.* New York: Vintage Books. (Original work published 1955)

Yeats, W. B. (1962). Among school children. In L. Untermeyer (Ed.), *Modern British poetry.* Orlando, FL: Harcourt Brace. (Original work published 1928.)

PART ONE

THEORY:
THE MEANING
OF WORK

CHAPTER ONE

The Spirit in Career Counseling

Fostering Self-Completion Through Work

Mark L. Savickas
Northeastern Ohio Universities College of Medicine

CAREER COUNSELING THAT envisions work as a quest for self and a place to nourish one's spirit helps clients learn to use work as a context for self-development. Career counseling that cares for the spirit seeks to identify how clients wish to spend their lives and which projects are worth their lives. This concern with passionate and spirited commitment to work goes beyond individual achievement and careerism to teach clients that work is a social activity, one in which they connect with, contribute to, and cooperate with other people. Using work in their quest for self involves more than just fitting themselves to an occupation's ability and interest requirements. The search for meaning involves meshing a life story with its preoccupations and projects into the communal effort to ensure survival and cultural self-realization for the group, not just individuals. To be fully alive means to share our unique contribution by joining spirit with other people in celebrating life through work, love, friendship, and worship.

This chapter begins with an explanation of how spirit moves a life and character charts its course. Attention then turns to how individuals can use work as a context for self-development and manifestation of spirit. The next section explicates how counseling that cares for the spirit can help clients use an occupation to become more complete. This is followed by a description of a career counseling model centered in client stories that show spirit. The next section discusses how to turn spirited preoccupations into social occupations. Finally, a concluding section asserts that occupational manifestations of spirit that produce individual achievements should in due course become social contributions.

SPIRIT, CHARACTER, AND MEANING

To be alive is to move. Our animation distinguishes us from inanimate objects and from rooted plants and at the same time shows the world who we are. *Spirit can be viewed as the activating force or essential principle that helps to give life to physical organisms.* The very origins of the word *spirit* arise from words denoting blow, breathe, and wind. A spirited person feels full of energy, enthusiasm, and courage. Individuals experience this spiritual courage as a sense of meaning that breathes life into situations. The passions, aspirations, frustrations, and anxieties that arise from meaning give life significance and chart its course. As an essential principle of life, spirit moves (or motivates) the individual and does so in a certain direction.

Spiritual courage orients most human beings to move in the same general direction. Individuals strive to become whole as they move from where they are to where they want to be. Adler (1956) identifies this direction as moving from a felt negative to a perceived plus. The perceived plus refers to improved adaptive capacity, not egocentric self-aggrandizement. Freud (1948) identifies the direction of development as "from it to I," which he labels the *ego paradigm*. Maslow (1954) refers to the principal direction of human movement as from gratifying biological needs to actualizing the self. In relating spirit to work, Miller-Tiedeman and Tiedeman (1985) refer to this movement as *career* or the imposition of direction on human life. The movement toward self-completion, regardless of what we call the signposts, increases adaptive capacity. Unfortunately the new capacities do not always get put to good use because some individuals invest their new skills in useless self-aggrandizement rather than useful contribution to others.

To have the spiritual courage to move forward, toward other people and community responsibilities, defines mental health. Of course, not everyone has the courage and the encouragement to move toward other people and embrace the common unity of life or community living. Lack of movement or movement toward material goals and extrinsic rewards such as power, prestige, and possessions tears the fabric of social living. In addition to interpersonal problems, individuals with stalled or misdirected movement experience intrapersonal demoralization, discouragement, and dispiritedness. In psychodiagnostic terms, stalled or hesitant movement can be called *neurosis*. Moving away from people can be called *psychosis,* whereas moving against people can be called *psychopathy*. Healthy people move toward the community of individuals because they realize that life involves connection between, contribution to, and cooperation with other people. As individuals move toward and with people, they quickly learn that their communal salvation and personal integration reside in the social roles proffered by the community.

Individuals enact life through social roles. Super (1980) identifies a rainbow of major life roles that include student, worker, citizen, leisurite, and family member. Adler (1956) believes that the three major roles are work, friends, and love. Cabot (1914) views the primary roles as work, love, play, and worship. Whatever personal tapestry of roles one weaves into a life pattern, the key role is work. Freud (1961) asserts that work is the basic tie to reality. Havinghurst (1954) agrees that work is the key role in life because it provides for money, association, structure, creativity, and self-expression. Other roles can offer the last four in his list, but work is unique in providing economic support. Erikson (1968) taught that work also provides personal and social identity. In stating occupational interests, individuals also state, in tangible terms, who they are and what they want.

Obviously the spiritual quest to become more complete, more whole, usually involves work. As a context for human development, work activities provide a venue for becoming more than one used to be. In and through work, individuals develop themselves by expressing the occupational interests, vocational talents, and work values that move them from a felt negative to the perceived plus. This progressive development constitutes a spiritual quest for meaning and self-completion that, in the process, helps people become someone they want to be, a person they themselves would like.

WORK AS A CONTEXT
FOR SELF-DEVELOPMENT

Work provides a major context in which individuals can meet their needs for agency and for union. Through work as a productive activity, people can be active agents who advance themselves and improve the world. Through work as a social contribution, individuals can share the fruits of their labor with family, friends, and neighbors. Through working with people, individuals can gratify their needs for cooperation and companionship. Thus work provides a forum for both individual identity and social significance. Accordingly, individuals can and do use work to develop into the self they want to become as well as manifest that self in social situations. Individuals both use and are used by work. Traditional career counseling emphasizes how employers and their occupations use the client's abilities and interests. Career counseling that attends to the individual's spirit, in addition, addresses how people can use occupations and work for personal and spiritual development. An occupation can allow people to resolve unfinished business from childhood, create meaning, advance life projects, and increase personal agency.

When counselors think of work as a theater to be used for developing the self, they want to know the manner in which a client seeks self-development and spiritual nourishment. Character sets the method of development. As architects of their own character, individuals choose their own style. Character is the personal mode of expression that individuals use to adapt to the world in which they live. Character is implemented in and made manifest through work. Motivational constructs explicitly denote the direction (or "perceived plus") that character implicitly sets. Remember, individuals are already animated, because to be alive is to move. Motivation does not move people; rather, it directs them. By providing a motivational direction, character charts the life course and channels daily behavior (Kelly, 1955).

Relative to the world of work, counselors focus on three modes of character expression: needs, values, and interests. These constructs point the direction in which clients think they can move to become more complete. Each mode deals with different aspects of motivation. Needs arise from a felt sense of incompleteness. Needs indicate the qualities that people lack yet think they require to feel secure and to become more whole. Values denote the objects or gratifications in the world that people seek to satisfy their needs. Values are general goals that confirm who we are and what we wish to become. They signal a commitment to a way of life. In addition, values are communal and consequential because, as community sanctioned ways to meet needs, they relate the individual to the community (Bruner, 1990). Interests bridge needs and goals. Needs explain the why of life movement, whereas values describe what the goals are. Interests propose the route that links the *why* of needs to the *what* of values. Interests state a preferred *how* and project specifically how individuals propose to attain the goals that satisfy their needs.

For example, a career counselor might display a strong need to nurture other people yet at the same time to control and dominate. She can gratify these opposing needs through pursuing altruistic values that guide her to actively promote the welfare of other people. She may be interested in doing this as a career counselor but also as a social worker, minister, or nurse because these professionals also tell people what is good for them. Notice that in this example the career counselor's needs for nurturance and dominance naturally lead to altruistic values that she implements in a social occupation. People who possess this type of integrated, coherent set of interconnected needs, values, and interests have an easier time establishing a clear and stable sense of identity: They know where they are and where they want to go. When individuals exhibit disjunction among needs, values, and interests, they usually encounter difficulty in resolving the identity crisis because they are overwhelmed by life problems and confused as to how to chart their life course.

RATIONAL VERSUS SPIRITUAL CAREER COUNSELING

Personal needs, work values, and occupational interests have become the objective indicators that individuals use to gauge their life projects. Counselors foster adolescent self-awareness as a foundation for career decision making by providing objective feedback to students about their needs, values, and interests. Occupational information pamphlets describe the profile of needs, values, and interests that characterize satisfied and successful workers in diverse occupations. Individuals are then encouraged to use "true reasoning" to match their motives to those required in different occupations and then select the most fitting match as their occupational choice (Parsons, 1909). This matching process itself can be assisted by objective techniques such as interest inventories. For example, in responding to the *Strong Interest Inventory*™ (Harmon, Hansen, Borgen, & Hammer, 1994), individuals report their interest in particular occupations, activities, hobbies, and types of people. A computer then matches this character profile to normative profiles of successful and satisfied individuals employed in many different occupations. The computer uses complex algorithms, or "true reasoning," to rationally indicate good matches between an individual and various occupations.

The objective, scientific, and rational methods of applied psychology do a fine job of representing common sense: They effectively and efficiently use actuarial methods to systematically match individuals to normative data (Super, 1954). The norms deal with aspects of character as an assembly of traits. Individuals' scores on each trait are graphed on a sheet of paper using a normal distribution or some variation of it. The individual learns, for example, that he or she scored at the 80th percentile on needs for nurturance and dominance and at the 70th percentile on altruistic values. This tells the person that his or her profile resembles those of people employed as career counselors. Objectively, the pattern of trait scores suggests that he or she is a fitting match for the profession of career counseling. Although effective, this rational approach usually ignores the essence of a client's unique character. What clients believe and feel about life is expressed in the unified, indivisible pattern that is more than its parts (i.e., assembly of traits). As Gestalt psychology asserts, the whole is greater than the sum of its parts. The best career counseling joins the individual's private sense about life and its meaning to the common sense through conversation and dialogue. When clients articulate their spirit, it becomes more coherent to them and clearer to their friends and neighbors as well.

People are so much more than the traits that personality and career inventories objectively measure and profile. An individual transcends all objective classification taxonomies. A person possesses a spirit. This spiritual dimension is how people experience themselves. Individuals organize their lives around specific meanings. They do not know themselves by their traits; instead they know themselves by their passions and purposes. This subjective "I" cannot be measured like the objective "me." It can be felt, understood, and communicated but not counted. The essence of a person, her or his unique spirit and activating force, can only be comprehended as a whole pattern, not trait pieces. In music, the melody is more than the individual notes. In life, the theme is more than behavior. The theme of a life gives it meaning and distinction, like the *ideé fixe* or leitmotif in a piece of music by Berlioz or Wagner. It is the life theme that makes the person self-consistent and therefore knowable to the self and recognizable by others. Even when the melody is transposed to another key, it is still identifiable because its essence remains; like a melody, a person cannot change if in some important sense she or he does not remain the same. Behaviors and strategies for living can change or be transposed as people mature, yet the core theme remains constant. Even as people elaborate and increase their repertoire of adaptive abilities and interests, they maintain a self through cohesiveness among and continuity in their needs and values.

THE SIGNIFICANCE OF STORIES

The empirical tradition of rational career counseling does not encompass complex human qualities such as spirit, consciousness, and purpose. Science examines parts; personal stories explain the whole. Stories tell us the situation, the needs, the goals, the interests, and the outcomes. It is through stories that counselors gain access to a person's spirit and life theme. The theme in a life story makes biography possible. Career counselors who wish to help people plot a life story, not just choose an occupational position, use the literary techniques of the biographer to identify the theme of the life story already in progress. Some career counselors have articulated these narrative means to therapeutic ends in writing about career as story (Jepsen, 1992), self-construction (Neimeyer, 1992), subjective experience (Savickas, 1993, 1995a, 1995b), and narrative (Cochran, 1990, in press). These authors strive to help clients become more active agents in authorizing and authoring their own lives. Their first step in facilitating life planning involves clients in identifying and articulating their spirit in terms of the theme that runs through their lives (Csikszentmihalyi & Beattie, 1979). Counselors do this by asking clients to look at themselves as the central character in a drama and then discover the pattern in their unfolding lives, give form to their identity, and imagine future scenes.

Career counselors who care for the spirit possess the ability to see patterns. Events that cannot be patterned are useless to the client. Counselors need the ability to recognize patterns because most clients cannot say who they are or articulate their life theme. The essence of people, their unique spirit and activating force, can be seen only in the whole pattern, not in the individual traits, but clients find it easier knowing and reporting their traits; they are so embedded in their own pattern that they do not realize they have one. They need increased self-awareness to know their life themes, the unique arrangement of life force that defines them. Even the few clients who grasp the essential principle that guides their lives find it difficult to articulate it explicitly.

What most clients have is an implicit and intuitive understanding of their life theme. Although they cannot readily report the theme, they can tell stories about their pain, preoccupations, and projects. Each person cares about some things more than others and feels passionate about only a few issues, which are preoccupations at the core of the spirit. The pattern is revealed as people tell stories about how they turned these private preoccupations into public projects. These stories usually concern defining moments in their lives, models who inspire them and nourish their spirit, and leisure activities that set their spirit free. It is in these stories that people know themselves best, because in them they store their experiences and digest the meaning of these experiences. Thus counselors can know their clients better through stories than through theories.

Finding Themes in Stories

Over the years, I have developed a method for identifying the life theme that activates and characterizes an individual. As a career counselor, I seek to help individuals turn their pain into progress. I aspire to help them transform their tensions into intentions, not pretention. The simple idea is to show them how to use the social role of work as a theater in which to advance their story, develop themselves, and become more whole. It is counseling focused on the whole rather than the parts. Unfortunately the whole is harder to see than the parts. Accordingly, most career counselors start their professional lives looking only at the parts. However, as they gain experience, counselors become more interested in what connects the parts, the pattern that makes everything else about the person meaningful.

The heart of my counseling model is to identify a life theme by comprehending how clients try to actively master what they have passively suffered. This is the essence of Freud's ego paradigm, which identifies the master motivation in life as turning externally imposed pain, or "it," into personal strengths, or "I." In turning *it* into *I,* the individual turns symptoms into strengths, and if given the opportunity the strengths can become social contributions. Adler (1956) calls this movement from symptom to strength moving from "a felt minus to a perceived plus." Art Linkletter talked about turning lemons into lemonade, and General MacArthur spoke of turning victims into victors. Possibly the most elegant statement of this paradigm was penned by Milton (1667/1940) in *Paradise Lost* when he described Lucifer's arrival in hell. Lucifer turned to his followers and said, "Our torments also may, in length of time, become our elements" (p. 33). The theme of a life story can be traced by examining how the individual turned symptoms into strengths, tension into intention, and torments into elements. To do this, I ask clients for stories that reveal their spirit. Character and its formation are made visible and become available for analysis through personal stories. Stories are modes of knowing that capture the richness, uniqueness, and complexity of what life means to a client. From these stories about their torments and elements, their preoccupations and projects, I look to find the theme.

If one truly believes that the whole is in every piece, any story a client chooses to tell the counselor would suffice. Nevertheless, there are certain stories that are easier for counselors to understand. It is these stories that I seek. I start career counseling by asking clients how I can be useful to them. I carefully write down their answer and continually remind myself of it as I listen to their stories. It is only when I can understand how this opening statement exemplifies the client's life theme that I am ready to help that client use work as a theater for self-development and as a context for actively mastering what she or he has passively experienced. After listening and responding to the opening statement, I explain briefly why I want their stories, then immediately proceed to ask for the first story.

Early Recollections

The first stories I elicit from clients deal with the time when they were making up their mind about life. These stories reveal the key elements of their life theme. Consider an analogy to explain this point. Imagine that you are standing outside of a community theater and someone runs up and begs you to join a play in progress. You agree to do so and ask her what part you are to play. In response, she says that there is no time to tell you and she pushes you center stage as the curtain rises for Act II. There you stand. Think for a moment what you would do. You could retreat by running offstage, look to the director for orders, do a monologue that ignores the other actors, avoid attention by hiding behind a prop, try to get others to follow your script, stand still and do nothing, or watch what the other actors do and try to fit in. As strange as this may seem, we have all been cast into this situation. When our parents brought us home from the hospital, Act II began. Before we arrived, the play was in progress. Stated differently, before the individual was the community. At about age three or four, children start to decide what life means to them. The natural way to begin to construct a life plan is to look to family members and try to fit into the ongoing story by scripting our unique contribution to it. Other less desirable solutions are to retreat offstage into psychosis, become dependent upon parental direction, develop a narcissistic monologue, shyly avoid attention by hiding behind fears and obsessions, psychopathically manipulate the other actors to fit our own script, or stand still and depressively do nothing.

In their family of origin, individuals begin to script their lives to address the torments they experience at home, in school, and around the neighborhood. Some pain hurts more than all others, and that problem becomes a preoccupation. Individuals become sensitive to this particular pain and spend their lives trying to turn it into a strength, compulsively reliving the seminal event or events. Hopefully, with each repetition, they take another step toward mastery. The strengths they accrue in actively mastering what they passively suffered become the talents, needs, values, and interests that they implement in choosing an occupation. Their mastery and movement to a perceived plus actually explain the origins of the adaptive capacities measured by personality and interest instruments as well as provide a window on the unique spirit and life theme that define an individual.

I start by asking clients to tell me three stories about their early childhood; in fact I ask them for the three earliest recollections (ERs) they can remember (McKelvie, 1979). These stories contain their blueprint for life, the essence of their spirit. To provide some practice at seeing life patterns, consider the ERs of four different clients. I choose these ERs simply because each occurred in a car. The first client remembered driving with her mother and grandmother during a violent thunderstorm. The thunder frightened her until her grandmother told her a beautiful story about lightning being God playing with a flashlight and thunder being the angels dancing. She was reassured and learned to enjoy hearing thunder. The second client reported going on an extended summer vacation with her parents. The drive was long and boring yet she enjoyed passing time by writing stories in a blank booklet her grandmother had given her for that purpose. The third client also remembered driving on vacation. She was dancing in the back seat and enjoying herself when her mother told her to sit down and be still. The fourth client remembered getting into the car parked in her driveway so they could go to church. She stated that her mother purposely slammed the door on her hand.

Could these four stories actually portray lifelong preoccupations, a sensitivity to certain torments, and motivation for particular projects? Try to guess at the preoccupation and life course for each of these clients. The client who heard the thunder became a counselor who uses narratives and humor to help clients deal constructively with their fears and problems. The client with the blank booklet writes science fiction novels. The client who was enjoined to sit still and do as she was told selected a nontraditional career for women, against her parents' directives, and as a pioneer she stands up for her rights and those of other females. The fourth client suffered great paranoia and found it difficult to establish herself in a career because she believed other people sabotaged her. She decided to leave the world of work to concentrate on being a good mother and church volunteer.

With practice, a counselor can quickly discern life themes from ERs, but that is not the goal of career counseling. Instead the goal is for clients to become aware of their life themes and decide how to nurture or redirect their life projects. One technique for helping clients to do this involves writing headlines. After I have elicited three ERs from a client, I explain that effective headlines for newspaper articles always contain an action verb. Remember, to be alive is to move. Accordingly, a good headline summarizes the action in the story. I then ask the client to write a headline for each ER. We collaborate until the client is certain that the headlines fit. These headlines contain the gist of the life theme and, when read in sequence, reveal the direction of movement. We will use these headlines later when we discuss how to extend the life theme into the future and turn private preoccupation into public occupation.

In reading the three headlines, both individually and as a three-part sequence, the counselor can see the client's chief preoccupation and blue-print for life. The question becomes how to turn preoccupation into occupation, problem into opportunity, and symptom into strength. There are many possible methods for doing this, but I prefer a simple one—asking the client whom they admire.

Role Models

Of course, it is easy to see the connection between preoccupation and occupation in retrospect. But the career counselor's job is to see life prospectively, to extend a life theme into the future and forecast how pre-occupation can become occupation. I find that stories about admired peo-ple reveal clients' goals (values) as well as their preferred methods (inter-ests) for attaining these goals. If I can know only one thing about a person, I want to know whom she or he admires. My rationale follows Spranger's (1928) assertion that we know people best by what they value. Although the counselor can recognize needs from ERs, the narratives about role models reveal goals and interests. Through narration of the past (ERs), life becomes meaningful, but through narratives of the future (role models), tomorrow becomes real.

People who are admired are called role models because others model their self-construction after these images. Role models show ways to devise and develop better solutions to problems. Models serve as templates that individuals use to design their own lives. By finding people to admire, indi-viduals find possible selves (Markus & Wurf, 1987). As individuals develop, they imitate the role models and strive to be like them. This role-playing leads, in due course, to the development of interests and skills.

Hanna (1994) describes this process well when she writes about one of her role models. This professor of political science learned from Wonder Woman the value of warm, loving communities, that "women can do any-thing if they stick together," and that "a woman could be in love and still retain her own identity" (p. E2). Interestingly, Wonder Woman was con-sciously designed by a psychologist, William Moulton (the inventor of the lie detector), as a role model for his daughter and other children, a super-heroine who showed that love is stronger than violence. Because not everyone looks at a role model the same way, it is important to ask clients why they admire particular people. Counselors cannot assume that everyone admires Wonder Woman for her empowering message; people find different messages in her stories. A case in point: One young man found Wonder Woman fascinating because of her invisible airplane. He later became a research scientist who worked on designing the stealth bomber.

Let us be clear that individuals have more than one role model, that they idealize and identify with many people. They take bits and pieces from several heroes and heroines as they construct themselves. Accordingly, I ask clients who are still constructing their identities to name three people whom they admired when they were growing up. They can name famous people, individuals they actually knew, or fictional characters. After clients name three role models, I ask them to describe each one in some detail and if possible tell a favorite story about each one. Finally I ask clients to tell me how they differ from each person they admire. This question sharpens the focus of their self-report.

Of course, counselors listen at several levels to client descriptions of role models. First they listen for the collection of traits that the client believes will help them address their preoccupation and become more complete. Second, counselors listen for the overriding commonality that connects these three figures and reveals the essential goal. And third, they listen for the aspects of the heroines and heroes that clients reject and do not find useful in their own lives. In short, counselors need to hear the clients' goals/values and methods/interests for reaching these goals.

Certainly many counselors will wonder about the validity of using role models for recognizing values and goals. Once as I was explaining my view of role models, a student in the front row exclaimed, "I always admired Mighty Mouse. Does that mean I want to be a rodent?" Not to be deterred, I asked her what she admired about Mighty Mouse. She responded that Mighty Mouse always rushed to crisis situations and resolved them. With that response, the class began to laugh. Neither she nor I knew why they were laughing, so I asked them. They pointed to the jacket hanging over the back of her seat. The sleeve had a paramedic patch on it. She blushed and said that she worked part-time as a paramedic and that her ambition was to be a counselor who specialized in crisis intervention.

A similar incident occurred at a counseling conference. As I was explaining how people use role models to design their lives, a man seated on the center aisle said that this seemed too simplistic and deterministic. Of course, I had to ask him whom he admired when he was growing up. He responded, "Robin Hood. Try to make something of that." Fortunately I did not have to. The individuals seated in his row began to laugh. They said he was their counseling center director and they were his seven merry men, although four were female. They explained that he even insisted that they attend the conference with him and sit together at this session. Of course, they were glad to add further stories connecting Robin Hood to the director's management style and daily life. After a few minutes, he said, "Enough. I have to reconsider this."

One's collection of role models is a collection of possible selves. At first, this collection of selves is not integrated or coherent. As individuals mature and deal with the identity crisis (Erikson, 1968), they fashion these highly selective images into a clear and stable personal identity. In due course, individuals translate their personal identities into cohesive and unique vocational identities. Career counseling that cares for the spirit pays particular attention to tightening this integration of possible selves before translating it into a viable and suitable vocational identity. The skills, interests, and attitudes that constitute character are what rational career counseling matches to possible occupations. A deeper approach to matching tries to identify occupations that implement and develop character itself. The job should manifest who individuals are and want to become.

Articulating the Theme

After hearing the needs reflected in ERs and the values reflected in role models, the counselor attends to connecting the two. The connection between these two points is the life theme, the line of movement the person has chosen for his or her life course. In the language of career counseling, this connection can be called *interests*. The word *interest* comes from two Latin words, *inter* and *est*, meaning *it is between* or *to be between*. Interests are not in *us*; they are in situations. Interests relate individuals to their context by connecting personal needs to environmental goals and communal values. Interests focus the quest for self because they reveal how the individual plans to become more complete and how he or she envisions using the world of work as a context for further development (Savickas, 1995a).

As a counselor begins to learn this technique for identifying interests and the individual's quest for meaning, it may be helpful to write the client's needs/symptoms/ERs on the left side of a blank piece of paper and write the role models and goals on the right. The blank space between the needs and values is reserved for brainstorming possible interests that connect the two. Filling in this blank space is what clients seek from career counseling.

From this perspective, interests are solutions to problems in growing up (Carter, 1940). New and richer narrative unity comes from connecting ERs to role models. The technique gets its validity the same way a novel does, by coalescing the particulars of a life around a coherent theme. The theme is an explanatory proposition that makes sense of the life. Coherence is enhanced when the theme explicitly connects the story's beginning (ERs) to its middle (role models). This connection clarifies choices and in so doing makes it easier for clients to decide on an occupation and then write the next chapter in their life story.

Example

Consider an individual who reports a defining moment in life as follows: She is an only child who spent her first nine years on crutches because of a defect in her left knee. Her father, on his death bed, told her that he was disappointed because he had no son to keep his name alive. This haunting story echoes through her life as she continually feels her father's disappointment. She wants to live her life in a way that resolves this issue, yet how can she keep his name alive? This question at least implicitly preoccupies her and intuitively guides her life choices. Of course, she cannot solve this problem as her father would have liked, yet there are numerous resolutions. She must, however, perceive these options in her environment.

As a teenager, she works as a waitress in a diner. Every day a man comes in for lunch. Eventually she learns that he owns a gym and is a famous weightlifter whose name is in the Weightlifters Hall of Fame. She finds that she can actively master her leg defect through weight training, and eventually she also masters her main preoccupation. She becomes the first woman inducted into the Weightlifters Hall of Fame and in this way makes her father's name live forever. The title to this story as it appeared in a local newspaper also provides an example of a good headline: "Lifting Her Name Up High" (Rosewater, 1994). Notice how weightlifting became her passion because it integratively addressed her torments about a defective knee, a disappointed dad, and societal sex roles.

CAREER COUNSELING
THAT CARES FOR THE SPIRIT

The basic paradigm for rational career counseling consists of translating a self-concept into fitting occupational titles (Parsons, 1909; Holland, 1985a). Clients seek a counselor's guidance in identifying work environments in which they will feel belongingness and co-workers will appreciate their contributions. At a deeper level, career counselors can discuss how work will nourish the client's spirit and implement the client's passion and projects. Counseling that narrates the client's life theme combines objective person-position matching with the subjective meaning created by the client's spirited quest for meaning.

Narration

A narration should retell the life in a way that fosters understanding of the origins and meaning of clients' life themes and their relevance for career development. The narration helps clients to understand themselves and engage in more purposeful action. It should help them impose direction on their vocational behavior by clarifying their goals and the means to reach them. The narration provides a character sketch, one that includes the client's "superobjective." Stanislavsky, in his system for teaching acting, emphasized that each character in a play has an overall objective that motivates all of her or his behavior throughout the play. This superobjective welds together all aspects of the role, and the actor must know that overall objective in order to create an integrated and purposeful character (Levin & Levin, 1992). The same holds true for career-counseling clients. In knowing their character by its superobjective, they can more purposefully impose direction on their career choices and vocational behavior.

By attending to the essential principle and spiritual passion that activate a client, the counselor can weave a story. The story begins with a recitation of the three headlines from the ERs accompanied by a narrative description of the client's principle preoccupations and how they direct a quest for meaning. The counselor should in most cases be rather candid in retelling the origins of the spirit in the client's character. In other words, the counselor should clearly articulate the pain or problem most frequently experienced by the client and give examples of how it repeats itself in various life episodes.

Having identified the client's preoccupation, the counselor continues the story by discussing how the client's role models actually portray solutions to the concerns. Role models are important not for what they accomplished in their own lives but for what they can accomplish in the client's life (Cobb, 1991). It is useful for clients to consider how the models selected directions for their own lives or, in the jargon of counseling, how they chose values and constructed meaning. The counselor can help clients understand how their role models provided cultural scripts for them to use as they designed their life pattern. For example, the weightlifter can come to explicitly understand how a solution to the problem of keeping her father's name alive was embodied in her role model, a Hall of Fame member. Her work as a weightlifter was more than interesting; it was a passion that embodied her spirit. It made her more whole, more complete, and more effective. In short, weightlifting made her more herself. All clients, upon leaving counseling, should clearly understand that they are the architects of their character. In authoring their own lives, they are both storyteller and story.

The counselor should make sure that the client understands the narrative. If the client does not understand it or disagrees with some details, then the counselor needs to seek the client's revisions. When the narrative does not suit the client, the counselor should encourage him or her to edit the narrative so that it does fit. The counselor's goal is to be useful, not right. Even errors in the initial narration can be useful if they are used to heighten understanding and focus on important nuances. Working together, client and counselor should come to some agreement about the origins and progress of the story line. To check that we have reached clarity and agreement, I ask clients to tell me something that happened today that exemplifies the preoccupation that we have just articulated. Most clients do this easily; after all, the whole is in every piece. This brief exercise also reinforces the client's belief in the ongoing importance of his or her life preoccupation.

Interests

At this point, the counselor has narrated the client's story. By focusing on the life theme, the counselor has described the client's needs and their origins as well as values and their meaning. It is now time to discuss interests, or how the client may proceed in the future. Naturally there are as many ways of approaching this topic as there are counselors. My approach is to describe the client's interests as solutions to personal pain or problems. Of course, I do this by describing how the person's talents and interests relate to his or her preoccupation as well as how these solutions should be implemented and made manifest in fitting occupations. In an ideal situation, work implements the self-concept (Super, 1961). Work can be a vocational manifestation of identity. This means that the life theme, with its vocational needs, work values, and occupational interests, finds autonomous expression in job activities. In turn, the work itself becomes a context for further development and greater mastery. Unfinished business from childhood can be addressed and old issues worked out in a new situation.

Identifying specific occupations for a client to explore flows seamlessly from the discussion of the client's life theme and its implementation in future roles. Work that interests the person is recognized because it already lies in the direction the individual is moving. Once the counselor knows the client's line of movement, the group of occupations the client may find interesting and useful is clearly circumscribed. The pattern of needs limits which values and interests can be useful to the individual. The inherent direction he or she has chosen shapes the occupational activities that can in due course attract his or her interest (Anygal, 1941). So the little girl who finds consolation and courage in her grandmother's story about God's flashlight later finds herself attracted to occupations in which she can listen to people's fears and encourage them with healing words of her own. We cannot easily predict whether she will be a social worker, nurse, counselor, psychiatrist, minister, or bartender, yet we know that she will carve out an occupational niche in which she can use the skills she has rehearsed these long years. Her social contribution comes in helping other people overcome their fears using the strengths modeled by her grandmother and rehearsed by her since she was a child. In this way, her preoccupation becomes her occupation and her spirit is engaged and nourished as she earns her daily wage.

The actual choice of specific occupations to explore is usually easy because clients have secret ambitions or occupational fantasies that show the way. Eliciting these expressed interests can be rather straightforward once the client has learned to trust and collaborate with the counselor. Simply asking clients what occupations appeal to them typically produces a good list with which to start. The first page of one of the most popular objective interest measures, *The Self-Directed Search* (Holland, 1985b), asks clients to list their occupational daydreams. According to empirical research, this page is the best section of the measure for predicting what occupation the individual will enter (Touchton & Magoon, 1977). A list of occupational daydreams can now be quite useful because the occupations have a context within the life theme. Examining the occupations listed with regard to their relevance to the client's needs and values, problems and solutions, tensions and intentions clearly reveals those occupations that merit in-depth exploration. This exploration typically uncovers a few additional occupations to explore, yet the expanded list retains a coherence and consistency that the client understands.

If the counselor does not want to ask clients about occupational daydreams or the client responds with only a few occupational titles, then there are alternative ways to generate a personally meaningful list of occupations for the client to explore. One easy way is to identify the client's vocational personality type (Holland, 1985a) by assigning typological codes to the ERs and role model descriptions provided by the client. It is usually pretty clear from the ERs and role models what objective code best describes the client's character. With this vocational personality type code, the counselor and client can scan *The Occupations Finder* (Holland, 1985c) to generate a list of occupational titles for client reaction and exploration.

If desired, the client could even generate a list of occupations to explore by taking an interest inventory such as the *Strong Interest Inventory* (Harmon, Hansen, Borgen, & Hammer, 1994). Again, however, in reviewing the results of the *Strong,* the counselor should interpret the scores in context of life themes so clients deeply understand why they scored high on certain occupations. Situating the scores in clients' life themes explains why a few occupations for which they earn high scores may not appeal to them. I recall one client who scored high on optometrist. It was the only high score in that occupational group. She had no attraction to the field and wondered how she resembled optometrists. I asked her if she would like to explore optometry to answer that question. She responded, "Absolutely not. I am not interested in that kind of work. How could it possibly show up on this test?" I suggested that we review her ERs. In her third ER, she reported a story in which the son of her mother's friend teased and chased her. She ran to her dog for protection, thinking the boy could not get close to her. In anger, he threw a rock that hit her in the eye. The two mothers took her into the bedroom to tend to her eye. Her headline was "Dog plan fails to control boy." I asked her if it could be that her sensitivity to eye injury may have been enough to make her score similar to optometrists, although she had no intent of becoming an eye doctor. She agreed. It appeared that the main preoccupation scripted in this ER dealt with how she would relate to men, not the world of work. In contrast, a man who was interested in optometry had as his second ER a story about being embarrassed when his first-grade teacher called him to the front of the class so that she could clean his dirty glasses. One difference between the two stories is that her ER dealt with eyes, whereas his ER involved eyeglasses.

FROM SOLUTION
TO SOCIAL CONTRIBUTION

By now it is clear that the client's personality is a solution, one that resolves problems in growing up and in so doing produces character. Career counseling that cares for the spirit does not end when clients understand how to turn preoccupations into occupations. It continues by focusing on how clients can use the solution to make a social contribution. Counselors approach the issue of social contribution by discussing how clients can use the work role as a context in which to further master their problems and to implement their life projects. However, I would like to go further and discuss the spiritual nourishment that comes from turning personal solutions into social contributions. It is too easy to get trapped in careerism, or egocentric uses of work, by focusing on personal victory (Richardson, 1993; Savickas, 1994). These personal victories can become social failures if they focus exclusively on the "three p's" of power, prestige, and possessions. The path to growth goes from symptom through strength toward social contribution. Strong people need to be generous, to share the solution with the community.

Counseling theorists, to a great degree, talk about themselves in their theories, turning their private victories into public gifts. Therefore consider, as an example of turning personal solutions into social contributions, the lives of three leading psychodynamic theorists. Sigmund Freud's self-analysis of the Oedipal triangle that enmeshed him remains one of the great intellectual achievements of the modern era. Through his self-analysis, Freud created *a* truth that freed him from his own neurosis. Had he stopped with this private victory in which he actively mastered what he passively suffered, society would never have heard of him. Fortunately Freud made a social contribution by sharing with Viennese society his newfound strength, thereby turning his personal solution into a form of therapy that remains helpful to individuals who suffer problems similar to those he experienced. Of course, his theory and therapy for dealing with sexual trauma by making the unconscious conscious have little relevance for individuals who suffer from different problems. Consider Alfred Adler, for another example. Adler's problems did not constitute a sexual neurosis. He envied and felt inferior to his older brother. Adler's solution was to develop the courage to cope with life's tasks and feel equal to other people. His solution became a social contribution in his theory of sibling rivalry, insights into birth order positions, and therapy that uses encouragement techniques to overcome feelings of inferiority. A third and final example comes from the life of Erik Erikson, who escaped Nazi Germany and struggled as a disoriented immigrant in his new country, the United States. When he actively mastered his disorientation and established his new identity and transformed life, he renamed himself from Erik Homberg to "Erik, son of myself," or Erikson. His new name symbolized the self-constructive process he had completed. Erikson shared his solutions and strengths as a social contribution in the form of a theory of psychosocial identity development. He explained that adolescents resemble immigrants to a new country, because they leave the land of childhood to explore the land of adulthood. As immigrants do, adolescents must cope by constructing an identity that achieves inner certainty and outer recognizability.

We could continue to describe each counseling theory as an extension of the theorist's active mastery of personal problems, but most readers are probably already familiar with the personal origins of their preferred approach to counseling. There may even be some truth to the speculation that counselors use theories that address their own preoccupations because it is so easy for them to learn these theories. In career counseling that cares for the spirit, counselors strive to help clients understand how they too can turn their private victories into social contributions.

CONCLUSION

Career counseling that cares for the spirit attends to both career and the person who constructs the career. By dealing with both the personal preoccupation and the public occupation, counselors help clients to manifest their spirit and character through work. Clients learn to use occupations as a context in which they can become more complete and continue to actively master what they have passively suffered. Counselors foster client development through nurturing the spiritual courage that propels clients to use work as a forum for turning their problems into their elements.

REFERENCES

Adler, A. (1956). *The individual psychology of Alfred Adler* (H. L. Ansbacher & R. R. Ansbacher, Eds.). New York: Basic Books.

Anygal, A. (1941). *Foundations for a science of personality.* New York: The Commonwealth Fund.

Bruner, J. (1990). *Acts of meaning.* Cambridge, MA: Harvard University Press.

Cabot, R. (1914). *What men live by: Work, play, love, and worship.* Boston: Houghton Mifflin.

Carter, H. D. (1940). The development of vocational attitudes. *Journal of Consulting Psychology, 4,* 185–191.

Cochran, L. (1990). *The sense of vocation: A study of career and life development.* Albany: State University of New York Press.

Cochran, L. (in press). *Career counseling as narrative construction.* Albany: State University of New York Press.

Cobb, W. (1991) Thought for the day in a daily calendar.

Csikszentmihalyi, M., & Beattie, O. V. (1979). Life themes: A theoretical and empirical exploration of their origin and effects. *Journal of Humanistic Psychology, 19,* 45–63.

Erikson, E. H. (1968). *Identity: Youth and crisis.* New York: Norton.

Freud, S. (1948). *Beyond the pleasure principle.* London: Hogarth.

Freud, S. (1961). Civilization and its discontents. In *Complete psychological works (Vol. 21).* London: Hogarth. New York: Norton. (Original work published 1930)

Hanna, M. (1994, March 29). A little girl's role model in the comics. *Cleveland Plain Dealer,* p. E-2.

Harmon, L., Hansen, J. C., Borgen, F., & Hammer, A. (1994). *Strong Interest Inventory manual* (5th ed.). Palo Alto, CA: Consulting Psychologists Press.

Havinghurst, R. J. (1954). Retirement from work to play. In E. Friedmann & R. Havinghurst (Eds.), *The meaning of work and retirement.* Chicago: University of Chicago Press.

Holland, J. L. (1985a). *Making vocational choices: A theory of vocational personalities and work environments* (2nd ed.). Odessa, FL: Psychological Resources Associates.

Holland, J. L. (1985b). *Self-directed search*. Odessa, FL: Psychological Resources Associates.

Holland, J. L. (1985c). *The occupations finder.* Odessa, FL: Psychological Resources Associates.

Jepsen, D. A. (1992). Understanding careers as stories. In M. Savickas (Chair), *Career as story.* Symposium conducted at the meeting of the American Association for Counseling and Development, Baltimore.

Kelly, G. A. (1955). *The psychology of personal constructs*. New York: Norton.

Levin, I., & Levin, I. (1992). *Working on the play and the role: The Stanislavsky method for analyzing the characters in a drama.* Chicago: Ivan R. Dee.

Markus, H , & Wurf, E. (1987). The dynamic self-concept. A social psychological perspective. *Annual Review of Psychology, 38,* 299–337.

Maslow, A. H. (1954). *Motivation and personality*. New York: HarperCollins.

McKelvie, W. H. (1979). Career counseling with early recollections. In H. A. Olson (Ed.), *Early recollections: Their use in diagnosis and psychotherapy.* Springfield, IL: Thomas.

Miller-Tiedeman, A., & Tiedeman, D. (1985). Educating to advance the human career during the 1980s and beyond. *Vocational Guidance Quarterly, 34,* 15–30.

Milton, J. (1940). *Paradise lost.* New York: Heritage Press. (Original work published 1667)

Neimeyer, G. (Ed.). (1992). Personal constructs in career counseling and development [Thematic issue]. *Journal of Career Development, 18*(3), entire issue.

Parsons, F. (1909). *Choosing a vocation.* Boston: Houghton Mifflin.

Richardson, M. S. (1993). Work in people's lives: A location for counseling psychologists. *Journal of Counseling Psychology, 40,* 425–433.

Rosewater, A. (1994, May 23). Lifting her name up high. *Cleveland Plain Dealer,* p. D-4.

Savickas, M. L. (1993). Career counseling in the postmodern era. *Journal of Cognitive Psychotherapy: An International Quarterly, 7,* 205–215.

Savickas, M. L. (1994). Vocational psychology in the postmodern era: Comment on Richardson (1993). *Journal of Counseling Psychology, 41,* 105–107.

Savickas, M. L. (1995a). Examining the personal meaning of inventoried interests during career counseling. *Journal of Career Assessment, 3,* 188–201.

Savickas, M. L. (1995b). Constructivist counseling for career indecision. *Career Development Quarterly, 43,* 363–373.

Spranger, E. (1928). *Types of men: The psychology and ethics of personality* (5th German ed.). (P. J. W. Pigors, Trans.). Halle: Max Niemeyer Verlag.

Super, D. E. (1954). Career patterns as a basis for vocational counseling. *Journal of Counseling Psychology, 1,* 12–20.

Super, D. E. (1961). Self-concepts in vocational development. In D. E. Super, R. Starishevsky, N. Matlin, & J. P. Jordaan (Eds.), *Career development: Self-concept theory.* New York: College Entrance Examination Board.

Super, D. E. (1980). A life-span, life-space approach to career development. *Journal of Vocational Behavior, 16,* 282–298.

Touchton, J. G., & Magoon, T. M. (1977). Occupational daydreams as predictors of vocational plans of college women. *Journal of Vocational Behavior, 10,* 156–166.

CHAPTER TWO

Creating One's Personal Meaning Throughout the Cycles of Life

Its Development in Career, Psychosocial, and Faith Realms

Beverly E. Eanes
Loyola College

The crisis of our time
As we are beginning
Slowly and painfully to perceive
Is a crisis not of the hands
But of the hearts.
  —*Archibald MacLeish*

MEANING IS A place in the heart. The crises that we experience today are a result of not first consulting the heart, for it sees more clearly than our intellect or our will. If, as Frankl (1969) states, our will is toward pleasure or power, then most of us who are of modern Western culture will find that something important seems to be missing in our lives. He also speaks of the "will-to meaning" as a primary force whose searching can only be fulfilled by each unique individual. Frankl thinks that God ordained a meaning for each of us to discover. In his book, *Man's Search for Meaning* (1963), Frankl states that striving for meaning was a primary force in his life as it was in the lives of others. Frankl notes that in Auschwitz, the prisoner who lost faith in his or her future was doomed, for the spiritual hold was also lost, which led to the physical and mental decline of the individual.

Frankl also believes that more than the meaning of life in general, meaning is specific for each person and specific to a given moment. To illustrate this point, he gives this example of posing just such a general question to a chess champion: "Tell me, Master, what is the best move in the world?" (1963, p. 172). Of course, the answer depends on who is playing and upon the position of each player in a particular game.

The therapist Irving Yalom (1980) considers that philosophers refer to two major categories of meaning. The first is terrestrial, which has to do with a specific person's life meaning and purpose. The second category of meaning is cosmic and refers to a spiritual ordering or design outside of the person. Each person must search for an individual meaning or coherence but at the same time identify with a connectedness to cosmic meaning.

In his book *The Phenomenon of Man,* Teilhard de Chardin (1959) speaks of cosmic coherence in which all of life is a single organism composed of all living things. Each individual shares in the enterprise and may thereby achieve a personal sense of meaning. Evolution moves as an orthogenetic process, a predetermined order with an invincible life ascent. De Chardin states, "Life, being an ascent of consciousness, could not continue to advance indefinitely along its line without transforming itself in depth" (p. 166). Love becomes part of this developmental ascent, as does the merging of the individual in spititual union with the cosmos.

Such meaning in one's life comes from reaching out to others in compassion. Matthew Fox (1979) writes that compassion "is the world's richest energy source" (p. xi) and is cosmic in its scope because of the true interdependence of all creatures. Truly reaching out to others in a meaningful way, however, is not possible without a place in the heart for one's own worth. Naylor, Willimon, & Naylor (1994), in *The Search for Meaning,* say that "without loving ourselves we cannot effectively search for meaning: 'Why should I try to find meaning for someone I don't even love?'"

(p. 186). How does one develop a healthy love of self and ultimately a search for meaning outside oneself?

Searching for meaning is a function of personality and as such is a life-long process, and there are constant challenges or crises that may disrupt or empower personality development. The importance of overcoming those obstacles can be seen in the child struggling to learn new tasks, and in that sense of accomplishment after a task is finally achieved. Or meaning can be found through relationships that are formed throughout our lives despite disagreements and heartaches. Also there is the meaning of satisfaction that often comes from service to others sometimes in simple ways, or through specialized skills learned after many years of education and training. Finally one can look back over one's life, at the end of that life, and feel that it was worthwhile, that a single individual can truly make a difference.

Whether one is struggling to move beyond psychosocial crises, finding a satisfying career path, or reaching out with faith beyond oneself, meaning is the essential component in all facets of life. Many theorists have looked at meaning, its origins, and its development, over the life span. This chapter concentrates on the ideas and the schema of three such theorists: Erik Erikson, Donald Super, and James Fowler.

ERIKSON: MEANING THROUGH THE LIFE SPAN

Meaning moves and develops over the life span primarily from a basic sense of trust of others, through to being able to trust in oneself, to being considered trustworthy, and finally to trusting God or a higher power even in the face of terrible struggles and ultimately death. As the child grasps for a handhold from the moment of birth, so too do we grasp for meaning to make sense of our world.

Erikson (1963) feels that meaning gradually evolves throughout a person's lifetime. In infancy, parents must "be able to represent to the child a deep, almost somatic conviction that there is a meaning to what they are doing" (p. 249). For the adolescent and young to middle-age adult, meaning is centered on establishing the self, creating a stable identity, developing intimate relationships, and achievieng a sense of mastery in professional endeavors. In mature adulthood, a person finds meaning in "self-transcendent ventures." In what Erikson calls the generativity stage, it becomes important to guide the coming generations whether or not it is one's own children or "in care and charity for the species."

Erikson gives equal weight to the psychological, biological, and social development dimensions of the emerging individuals. He states that a human being is involved at all times in all three processes of organization, somatic, ego, and societal (1963, p. 36). This interrelationship is crucial in order to make sense of the world. A brief look at Erikson's psychosocial stages reveals his sense of how meaning might develop as one moves through these turning points. Even though Erikson may not consider meaning in the sense of life's purpose until adolescence, experiences even in early childhood can impinge on the development of meaning.

Trust Versus Mistrust
(Birth to Eighteen Months)

Essentially the infant learns to trust through the trustworthiness of the mother or primary caretaker. It is the totality of the mother, the sights, sounds, and touching, to which the infant responds. Gradually the mother's response to the hunger pangs alone are not enough to satisfy the infant's needs. The child begins to look for her and then for her facial response, especially her smile. In this sensorimotor stage, it is almost as if the body becomes convinced that what it is doing has meaning. Being nourished and cherished by the parents, the infant feels an inner sense of trust for the meaning of the parents' reponses. Erikson feels that it is the quality of the relationship and not the quantity of caretaking tasks that demonstrates love to the infant. The quality "combines sensitive care of the baby's individual needs and firm sense of person trustworthiness within the trusted framework of their culture's lifestyle" (1963, p. 249). It is through this process that the child forms a sense of identity and later becomes someone trustworthy to herself and to others.

The infant also responds, when something causes the mother to become tense or anxious, by fussing or crying. The mother will in turn respond to her offspring with more tension. In all of Erikson's stages, there must be a balance between positive and negative components, and in infancy the balance is between trusting and mistrusting, with trusting being predominant. For instance, a child is increasingly able to tolerate mother's absence without crying when a consistent pattern is established: that the mother returns when needed. To Erikson, this was the infant's "first social achievement" (p. 247). Mother has become a certainty within the child as well as an external predictability. The meaning that is established in the primary relationship with the parent is an important stepping stone to the next set of psychosocial tasks. The hopeful meaning for the child who will begin to search for wider acceptance beyond the family seems to be, "Like my mother, people are basically good and trustworthy, but at times I need to be cautious."

Autonomy Versus Shame and Doubt (Eighteen Months to Three Years)

Erikson agrees with Freud that the focus at this stage is the anal zone. With the concomitant muscular development, there is a preoccupation with a physical holding on and letting go. At the same time, there is a desire to return to the infancy dependence while also wanting to assert oneself and eventually reach autonomy, described as an awareness of being, as separate from parents. These simultaneous conflicts can lead to either constructive or destructive modes of existing. There can be cruel restraint or holding as in loving nurturance, just as there can be unleashed destructive forces or letting be what will be in a relaxed manner. The child tests the limits between holding on and letting go, and until the child develops discretion, the parents need to be consistently reassuring and yet open to the trials that must be attempted. The shame referred to in this stage is a self-consciousness, and Erikson (1963) felt that it was "essentially rage turned against itself" (p. 252). The doubt comes from a fear of failure, particularly related to regulating the anal sphincter and the appropriateness of the time and place in which the product is left behind. Self-control can have lasting effects in self-esteem and pride, whereas shame and doubt can develop from and continue to be a fear of overcontrol by others.

Successfully moving through this stage comes from the child having trust in himself, which develops from the previous stage as well as through parental guidance in this stage. This guidance includes allowing the child movement toward more independence within needed safety limits. Balance for the child needs to be toward flexibility with self and others. Meaning comes with free choice and yet some self-restraint.

As an example, picture the two- or three-year-old standing at the side of the swimming pool showing both her eagerness and trepidation as the parent, waiting in the pool, reaches forward to catch the child when she jumps. After several false starts and much reassurance that the parent will catch her, she lets go of the solid surface beneath her feet and splashes down into the waiting arms. Trust was essential for the child to even consider letting go, and now she is ready to do it all over again, but not with someone she doesn't know.

Initiative Versus Guilt
(Three to Six Years)

At this stage, there is a great deal of curiosity, and the child searches with imagination and self-confidence. The child at this age is very loving, and there is much play activity that includes choosing meaningful toys. From observation and play, the child learns about roles and purpose in life. He or she seems to have boundless energy, and usually mistakes are forgotten quickly. Erikson (1963) writes, "Initiative adds to autonomy the quality of undertaking, planning and 'attacking' a task for the sake of being active and on the move" (p. 255). Some fantasies can be consuming and lead to anxiety. The child makes a final bid as the favored one with the mother, and boys may suffer fear of castration for indulgence in these fantasies. The child may be afraid to take risks for fear of making mistakes or increasing guilt as opposed to being eager for new tasks. Erikson speaks about the "fateful split . . . between potential human glory and potential total destruction" (p. 256). The split is between the growth-producing exuberant self and the parental self that observes and punishes. The child may see self as bad or may have been told so by others, and this will restrict his or her movements. The child develops a conscience, and meaning comes with learning about his or her purpose in life.

Industry Versus Inferiority
(Six to Twelve Years)

The child is now eager to learn how to do and make things with others, which leads to the capacity for work enjoyment. She or he finds that enthusiasm and curiosity are tempered by the need to learn culturally specific technology. In fact, recognition comes when the youngster produces something useful. The at-risk child is the one who does not receive recognition for his or her efforts. He or she may develop a sense of inferiority and inadequacy.

Though nursery school and kindergarten may precede this stage, at this time children make the main transition from the family into society. However, "many a child's development is disrupted when family life has failed to prepare him for school life, or when school life fails to sustain the promises of earlier stages" (Erikson, 1963, p. 260). Meaning comes with learning specific skills related to the child's work purpose in life, especially in concert with others.

Identity Versus Identity Confusion (Twelve to Twenty Years)

It is in these adolescent years that the developmental tasks are to integrate childhood identifications, biological drives, and social role opportunities. There is concern for how one appears to others in dress, actions, and achievements. Adolescents identify with heroes and cliques and exclude those who seem different from themselves. They try out various roles while asserting independence and reexamining values. There is a need for continuity in what one means to others, which gives the adolescent a sense of ego identity.

A heart-wrenching yet inspiring story of a teenager appears in a newspaper article, *The Big Brother* (Leyden, 1996): James Holling is sixteen, and for two years he has freely chosen to spend his time outside of school caring for his younger sister, who has a serious and possibly incurable illness. Though his path is more complicated than most, and though he has found a special meaning in his life, he is nonetheless an adolescent. Leyden writes,

> Here is what it is like to be a 16-year-old boy. Life is perfidy. Your voice betrays you. Your body betrays you. Your appetites betray you. You want to be yourself, if only you could figure out who that is. You are big and little. Strong and weak. Fearless and frightened. Your eyes meet the eyes of adults then shyly grope the floor. You are ungainly in body and soul. (p. F4)

Adolescents eventually are able to identify with their own sex and become comfortable being with the opposite sex. Due to the physical and psychological upheaval of these years, it is normal to have temporary role diffusion, but if it continues, people are unable to derive any satisfaction from activities and suffer from an overpowering sense of shame, isolation, and mistrust. Meaning comes when adolescents develop a philosophy of life and see themselves as true to their place in society and/or true to a person.

Intimacy Versus Isolation
(Twenty to Thirty-Five Years)

In young adulthood, individuals are able to establish intimacy with self (that is, with their inner life) and with others. They are able to accept their own potential, gifts, and ideas and then reach out in a committed way to others in friendship, love, and sexual fulfillment. Both ego and body must now be able to master conflicts and "face the fear of ego loss in situations which call for self-abandon: in the solidarity of close affiliations, in orgasms and sexual unions, in close friendships and in physical combat, in experiences of inspiration by teachers and of intuition from the recesses of the self" (Erikson, 1963, pp. 263–264).

Avoiding experiences of intimacy or of the readiness to isolate that Erikson (1963, p. 264) calls *distantiation,* which also may mean destroying those who threaten one's "territory," is the danger in this stage and a source of character disorders. Isolated people cannot enter into a committed relationship because they fear loss of self. Without intimacy, they lack a certain meaning, which normally has benefits both personally and for the wider society.

Generativity Versus Self -Absorption
(Thirty-Five Years to Retirement)

Erikson (1963) considers this the central stage for generativity; it "encompasses the evolutionary development which has made man the teaching and instituting as well as the learning animal" (p. 266). In middle age, one is willing to share one's work knowledge by guiding another because one recognizes the needs of self and others. It is important to be needed, and meaning comes with passing on one's virtues, hopes, and wisdom. Thus one becomes a caregiver in the wider social system.

Without this generativity, people become self-absorbed and stagnate. They regress to an earlier time of indulgence and may even develop a psychological or physical invalidism.

Integrity Versus Despair
(Retirement Years)

Older adults are able to gain more perspective about self and humanity. They have adapted to the disappointments as well as the triumphs of generative activities. They continue to be productive in some area of their life.

As Erikson (1963) says, only in this person "may gradually ripen the fruit of these seven stages" (p. 268). In this last stage, there is the fullest development of trust, and one who trusts does not fear death. The despairing person not only fears death but is also disgusted with life and bemoans what life has failed to provide. He or she feels cheated because there is no time left to try an alternate path.

Meaning in a life of integrity is the result of a personal philosophy that transcends the individual, uniting generations of humankind.

SUPER: MEANING THROUGH CAREER AND PERSONALITY DEVELOPMENT

Donald Super's theory is a developmental and longitudinal approach to career choices over the life span. He labels his approach as differential-developmental-social-phenomenological psychology because he attempts to unify these perspectives of psychology with certain aspects of career development (1969). Central to his theory is the integral confluence of personal development and career development.

Super (1990) defines career as "the life course of a person encountering a series of developmental tasks and attempting to handle them in such a way as to become the kind of person he or she wants to become" (pp. 225–226). He uses the phrase *career maturity* to describe the cognitive and affective processes involved with an individual's ability to cope with these developmental tasks imposed not only by biological developments but also by the expectations of society. Super speaks in terms of developmental stages. However, his theoretical development has gone through several revisions, but the major stages remain: growth, exploration, establishment, maintenance, and decline. The exploration stage can be further subdivided into the phases of fantasy, tentative, and realistic; and the establishment stage can be subdivided into the trial (committed) and stable phases. It is important to note that there are minicycles that occur when there is a transition from one stage to another or when there is destabilization due to outside socioeconomic or personal forces.

Super's Life Career Rainbow (1994), a life-span and life-space model, details the way in which the various roles we play evolve and intersect across the life span. Most people play nine major roles during their life, and these roles usually develop in chronological order from child, to student, to leisurite, to citizen, to worker (whether or not the person is employed), to spouse, to homemaker, to parent, and lastly to pensioner. Most commonly, work, home, school, and community are the theaters in which the roles are played. Herr and Cramer (1996) state, "It is in role shaping, redefining the expectations of others and of the role itself with one's conception of it, as well as in the choice of positions and roles, that the individual synthesizes personal and situational role determinants" (p. 236). The several roles that one plays can be played in more than one theater at a time, and each role affects the others. These various roles can either facilitate or be detrimental to one another. The sequential combination of these roles establishes the person's life space. However, as Super (1994), himself states about the Rainbow, "in seeking to deal adequately with the life span and life space, it merely *suggests* the situational and personal determinants of career" (p. 67). He sought to remedy this with the Archway of Career Determinants, a model showing the segmental aspects of his theory.

Blustein and Noumair (1996) write about the importance of context in the formation of the self and identity. They emphasize relational as well as cultural factors as important aspects of context. They feel that as the demands on one's work tasks become more intense, more interactions are needed between the individual's self and the social contexts. Therefore "the career realm represents perhaps one of the more important arenas in which to consider a more context-based concept of the self and identity" (p. 436). Super takes the social and cultural context into consideration in furthering his career models.

Super's Archway of Career Determinants (1994) was designed to depict the psychological characteristics of the person as well as societal influences and how each acts upon the other. The determinants are depicted by columns that support an arch representing the determinants' outcomes. The underlying structure for the columns is the biographical-geographical foundation of human development. There is an emphasis on the self, the person who is the keystone of the arch, who, through decision making, reflects the synthesizing of personal and social forces as they become organized into self-concepts as well as roles in society.

Super feels that this model is important in the way it portrays the systematic contribution of these elements to career development. The person weighs all of these factors when making career decisions. To Super, learning theory is what cements all of these segments together.

Life satisfaction and work satisfaction are dependent on the person find-ing "adequate outlets for abilities, needs, values, interests, personality traits, and self-concepts" (Super, 1990, p. 208). For most people, an occu-pation provides a focus for their lives and their personality, whereas for others the focus may shift during their lifetime.

In a Ladder Model of Life-Career Stages and Tasks, Super depicts the sequence of life stages, including the tasks and the typical ages in the var-ious stages and at the various transition points. It is important to note that though one is generally climbing the ladder, the ascent may at times be dis-continuous, especially in relation to a career. Such changes may bring dis-couragement and/or lead to greater satisfaction and meaning. For women with families, establishment may have to be revisited as reestablishment after children are in school or leave home.

Because the sequence in career as well as life development is rarely con-tinuous, Super (1990) developed a Cycling and Recycling Model for Developing Tasks. This model stems from the Ladder Model and shows how one cycles and recycles, or how one essentially faces the same devel-opmental tasks, which present themselves in different forms as one moves through life.

The need for satisfaction in work would seem to be a universal phe-nomenon that incorporates the heart of the self-concept. This personal meaning derived from one's work can have important implications, espe-cially as one reaches out into the community in service to others.

FOWLER: THE JOURNEY OF MEANING THROUGH FAITH

James Fowler also felt that the degree of self-concept implementation would lead to a proportional degree of work satisfaction as well as give meaning to the whole of our lives, especially within the context of faith. He states (1980) that faith is "a human universal," a generic journey, but one that is not completed by everyone: "Faith has to do with the making, main-tenance, and transformation of human meaning. It is a mode of knowing and being. In faith we shape our lives in relation to more or less compre-hensive convictions or assumptions about reality. Faith composes a felt sense of the world having character, pattern, and unity" (p. 53). We tend, of course, to think of faith in a religious sense, though Fowler sees faith more as "a way of leaning into or meeting life" (p. 54) that may or may not be religious in nature.

Faith develops from a foundation of relationship and trust in another. This is the basic trust resulting from the loving consistency of the infant's primary caregiver, which we have already discussed in regard to Erikson's developmental stages. As infants, we form a connection when we rely upon another and with faith become attached and committed. This commitment later reaches out to include others as well as ideals such as truth, justice, and duty. Commitment is also seen in marriage and the family and in striving for excellence in one's career.

Fowler (1981) states that faith is "the broadest and most inclusive relationship" in which the self relates to meaning, "the ultimate environment" (p. 56). This ultimate environment is symbolically expressed as the "Kingdom of God" by Jews and Christians, who relate to God as their central value and unifier. Faith, according to Fowler, involves a transformation in knowing beyond "the logic of rational certainty . . . integrated with and contextualized by a logic of conviction . . . faith is a core process in the total self-constitutive activity that is ego" (p. 64).

Over several years, Fowler, his associates, and his students interviewed 380 subjects of all ages and backgrounds, trying to understand how people make and maintain meaning in their lives. The results of their research led to the formulation of seven developmentally related and structurally distinct stages. These faith stages range from the primal or undifferentiated faith of the infant to the very rare universalizing faith.

Primal or Undifferentiated Faith (Infancy)

The infant becomes disposed to the world, though unconsciously, as he learns to trust or not to trust his early caregivers. Though the child is prelinguistic and preconceptual, the consistency of meeting somatic needs (and perhaps the spontaneity of play) leaves a lasting impression of promise and the lack thereof leads to a feeling of deprivation and abandonment. Though Fowler considers this to be a pre-stage, what the infant experiences is foundational to later faith development. "Primal faith arises in the roots of confidence that find soil in the ecology of relations, care, and shared meanings that welcome a child and offset our profound primal vulnerability" (Fowler, 1984, p. 53).

Intuitive-Projective Faith
(Two Years Old)

Language now becomes involved in mediating one's relations with others. Mind and body now wander freely. "Perception, feelings, and imaginative fantasy make up children's principal ways of knowing—and transforming—their experiences" (1984, p. 54). They are able to construct long-lasting images as they bring together wonder and meaning into their world. Stories and symbols of their faith traditions help them to understand God, especially in relation to their losses.

It is important to consider the transitions from one stage to another as "a successive progression of more complex, differentiated, and comprehensive modes of knowing and valuing . . . and significant alterations . . . in the basic orientation and responses of the self" (Fowler, 1984, p. 57–58). Most importantly, when speaking of faith stage transitions, it is the very essence of life meanings that are at stake.

The transition to the next stage comes when the child needs to know what is real and what is not so concrete. This is when operational thinking begins to emerge. Usually at this time, Oedipal issues are either resolved or submerged.

Mythic-Literal Faith
(Six to Seven Years Old)

Attitudes, moral rules, beliefs, and stories are incorporated within the child as symbols that indicate belonging to the family's community of meaning. These symbols are as yet literal and one-dimensional. With "stable categories of space, time, and causality . . . the world becomes more linear, orderly, and predictable" (Fowler, 1984, p. 55). While in the previous stage, the child was egocentric where another's perspective was concerned; now the child is able to recognize and take another's perspective.

As stories display contradictions, the child begins to reflect on meanings and to question the conflicts. The transition comes about through the use of formal operational thinking. And, as interpersonal sharing develops, so too does the need to connect in a personal way with the ultimate environment.

Synthetic-Conventional Faith
(Typically Early Adolescence)

It is possible that some adults may not move beyond this stage. Many spheres outside of the family call for attention, such as peers, school, and work, and sometimes even religion. Faith needs to bring together disparate information and values into a unifying outlook and identity. The synthesis is deeply felt, and though this worldview is somewhat unique to the individual, it nonetheless is derived from the beliefs and values of significant persons. This synthesis is tacit, rather than explicit, as critical self-reflection has not taken place.

The transition to the next stage comes about when there are serious clashes with valued sources of authority, such as when a church's edict is changed.

Individuative-Reflective Faith
(Late Adolescence or Adult)

Moving to this stage is critical as it is necessary for the individual to take the responsibility for his or her beliefs and commitments in a more explicit manner. One cannot escape the tensions that exist between the needs of self and those of society. For some people, this stage may not emerge before the mid-thirties to forties. Fowler (1980) sees a "double development" in this stage. The "self (identity) and outlook (worldview) are differentiated from those of others" and affect responses and interpretations that one makes (p. 72). There is a "demythologizing" at this stage as symbols are translated into conceptual meanings.

As one becomes ready for the transition to the next stage, one begins searching for something new, as deeper voices and images beckon beyond the logical distinctions and concepts of this present stage.

Conjunctive Faith
(Usually Mid-Life and Beyond)

This stage of faith involves "the integration of elements in ourselves, in society, and in our experience of ultimate reality that have the character of being apparent contradictions, polarities, or at the least paradoxical elements" (Fowler, 1984, p. 64). The boundaries, which from the previous stage seemed so firm, now become more permeable as one is more humbly aware of the role that the unconscious plays in our behavior. Death also takes on a greater reality as well as the increasing disabilities of age. God is more mysterious and yet more vital and important. "Doing the will of God . . . is something like creating a play together . . . our responses, our initiatives . . . as we try to shape our dance in relation to God's movements" (p. 67).

There is a commitment to justice and to the nourishment of others, cultural identity and meaning, an imperative of "an inclusive community of being" (Fowler, 1980, p. 73). There is a division, however, between a transforming vision and a world that has not been transformed, and one can become immobilized by one's compassion for that world. In rare instances, the division gives way to the radical actualization of universalizing faith.

Universalizing Faith

For universalizing faith to occur, two tendencies must be completed: radical decentration from self, which comes from really "knowing" people and faiths that are quite different than one's own; and valuing and valuation. The heart rests on centers of value that confer people's identities. These rare persons see the ultimate environment as "inclusive of all being. They become the incarnators and actualizers of the spirit of a fulfilled human community" (Fowler, 1980, p. 73–74). Their contagious nature and commitment to the source of their power can unify, liberate, and transform. They may die for their beliefs, which are often seen as subversive. They may also be seen as very lucid and endowed with a special grace and at the same time very human.

What can we learn from these three theorists about creating one's personal meaning throughout the life cycle? The specific components of each theory give us different perspectives on how the impact on life's meaning dovetails at important life junctures. This can be seen in the chart "Stages and Development in Career, Psychosocial, and Faith Realms," depicting the schema of all three theorists, as seen in Figure 1.

For a person to have meaning in life, he or she must be able to move through the crises at each stage of development and evolve toward the final integrity, have worthwhile work, and be sustained by a faith that reaches beyond the self. We face crises and challenges and need to make necessary choices at each life transition within our sociocultural context.

CHALLENGES AND CHOICES
LEADING TO MEANING

The earliest developmental challenges begin in utero, carry through the birth transition, and continue throughout one's life. From conception until death, the environment in which the organism exists is crucial. One's

	Donald E. Super *Career Stages*	Erik H. Erikson *Psychosocial Stages*	James W. Fowler *Stages of Faith*
Death		*Death*	*Death*
Old Age			
Late Adult	Decline (65 & over) — Retirement or Specialization/ Disengagement Deceleration (60–70)	Integrity vs. Despair (retirement years) "wisdom"	Stage VI Universalizing (Rare)
		Generativity vs. Stagnation (35–retirement) "care"	Stage V Conjunctive (Middle Adult & Beyond)
Middle Adult	Maintenance (45–65) — Innovation or Stagnation or Updating Holding (45–50)	Intimacy vs. Isolation (20–35) "love"	Stage IV Individuative-Reflective 20s & 30s (Young Adulthood)
Young Adult	Establishment (25–45) — Stable/Trial (Committed) Trial (18–25)	Identity vs. Role Confusion (12–20) "fidelity"	Stage III Synthetic-Conventional (Adolescence)
Adolescent	Exploration (14–25) — Tentative (14–18) Capacities (13–14)	Industry vs. Inferiority (6–12) "competence"	Stage II Mythic-Literal 6 Years to Adolescence (School Years)
		Initiative vs. Guilt (3–6 Years) "purpose"	Stage I Intuitive-Projective 2 Years to 6 Years (Early Childhood)
Child	Growth — Interests (11–12) Fantasies (4–10) Curiosity	Autonomy vs. Shame & Doubt (18 mos.–3 yrs.) "will"	
		Trust vs. Mistrust "hope"	Primal Faith (Undifferentiated Faith)
Birth		*Birth to 18 months*	*Birth to 2 years (Infancy)*
	Adapted from Super (1990, 1994)	Adapted from Erikson (1959, 1963, 1968)	Adapted from Fowler (1981, 1984)

FIGURE 1   Stages and Development in Career, Psychosocial, and Faith Realms

physical endowment alone does not determine the course of one's life. It is the sociocultural context in which we live, coupled with genetic endowment, that affect our growth and maturation. The challenges and choices with which we are confronted flow from this. Though the newborn may need only warmth and nourishment including nurturance to grow, as he or she does grow, the kinds of nourishment needed and received (or not received) become more complex. It is in the interaction between self and society that personal, spiritual, and career development take place.

In Erikson's first psychosocial stage, primal faith is shaken in the child who does not learn to trust. This generally occurs when the parent is not trustworthy. The infant who hungers for the nearness and consistent nurturance of a caring parent gives up when inconsistency and carelessness are the norm. Parents who provide less than consistent care risk not only safety, but the extinction of curiosity in their children.

Moving positively through each successive stage of development is dependent on accomplishing the developmental challenges and choices of the preceding stage. Therefore, career development and faith development rest on the fulcrum of psychosocial development. The child's primal undifferentiated faith turns to intuitive projective faith when, through trust, hope is instilled and curiosity spurs growth in all areas of development.

The autonomous initiating child will fantasize about the world of work, about becoming another Cal Ripken, Monica Seles, or Shaquille O'Neal—nothing is impossible or out of range. Similarly the child's notion of deity is unbounded by reason. God exists to protect the child from harm, but the child exists to be a friend to God and to keep the deity from getting too lonely.

The crisis of identity comes with adolescence. In the career area, fantasy gives way to interest and capacity and finally to tentative choice and trial occupations. Purpose leads to competence. "What can I really do?" and "What can I do that I like to do?" are the questions the adolescent and young adult ask. Friendship with the deity depends on successive and successful resolution of serious value clashes with all authority.

It is at this point that the quest for meaning in life begins to escalate exponentially. Before the identity crisis is resolved, the young adult must win the battle with role confusion. It is only when the battle is won that young adults can find intimacy and lasting love in family, direction and commitment in work, and a faith that is individuative and reflective.

Resolution of the self in these areas does not occur instantaneously but rather over a period of fifteen to twenty years. The challenges of adulthood are so many!

The horrors of violence on the street, the potential of global war, the trauma of death and despair, the threat of economic chaos—all of these keep adults teetering on the edge of meaningless. What is it really all about, one asks, if one lives only to die, wins only to lose at a later time, gains only to give up or give in? The powers of greed and uncaring constantly threaten generativity, and one learns painfully that meaning is illusive. It is especially so when one concentrates on acquiring instead of caring, and having power over others instead of sharing.

Furthermore, meaning eludes those who are alienated from others or from their inner selves in such a way that it becomes impossible to connect in community or in a one-on-one relationship (Naylor, Willimon, & Naylor, 1994). For such a person, the maintenance stage of career is stagnation, or at best, mere holding on.

Innovation and creativity, a freshness of appreciation, characterize generative adults who care about others and share with them their wealth of knowledge, goods, and aesthetic enjoyment. For those people, the main-tenance stage of career is exciting! Each day is a new opportunity. The contrast between generativity and stagnation demonstrates that the spiritual crisis of middle adulthood is nothing less than the eternal battle of love versus death.

CONCLUSION

It is by overcoming the threat of nonbeing through loving relationships with others, and through the sharing of one's gifts, that one is moved beyond individuative-reflective faith, and even beyond the conjunctive faith by which we integrate the diverse elements of self. The fully integrated adult can recognize not only that "humankind is my kind" but also that beyond job, the big career is life. This person is free to engage and disengage from work and ultimately from loved ones and from life itself. At the end of such a life, there may be sadness, but not despair, because the person of integrity knows that each human is mortal, but the Earth and its fullness will live on. Many people believe that they will live on beyond earthly boundaries, and perhaps will also be remembered here on Earth as a result of their love and their labors. It is the nature of humankind to labor. But ultimate meaning through human work is achieved only when people work to dispense both justice and mercy to all, so that both the beauty and the goods of the earth can be shared by all. This is the pinnacle of human development, the point at which universalizing faith and work are one.

REFERENCES

Blustein, D. L., & Noumair, D. A. (1996, May/June). Self and identity in career development: Implications for theory and practice. *Journal of Counseling and Development, 74*, 433–440. (Reprinted from *The phenomenon of man*, by P. Teilhard de Chardin, 1959, New York: HarperCollins.)

de Chardin, P. T. (1959). *The phenomenon of man*. New York: HarperCollins. (B. Wall, trans.).

Erikson, E. H. (1963). *Childhood and society* (2nd ed.). New York: Norton.

Fowler, J. W. (1980). Faith and the structuring of meaning. In C. Brusselmans (Convener) & J. A. O'Donohoe (Co-Convener), *Toward moral and religious maturity* (First international conference on moral and religious development). Morristown, NJ: Silver Burdett.

Fowler, J. W. (1981). *Becoming adult, becoming Christian: Adult development and Christian faith*. San Francisco: Harper San Francisco.

Fowler, J. W. (1984). *Stages of faith: The psychology of human development and Christian faith*. San Francisco: Harper San Francisco.

Fox, M. (1979). *A spirituality named compassion and the healing of the global village, Humpty Dumpty and us*. San Francisco: Harper San Francisco.

Frankl, V. (1963). *Man's search for meaning: An introduction to Logotherapy* [Special edition]. New York: Washington Square Press.

Frankl, V. (1969). *The will to meaning: Foundations and applications of Logotherapy*. New York: World.

Herr, E. L., & Cramer, S. H. (1996). *Career guidance through the lifespan: Systematic approaches* (5th ed.). New York: HarperCollins.

Leyden, L. (1996, Sept. 22). The big brother. *Washington Post*, F1, F4. F5.

Naylor, T. H., Willimon, W. H., & Naylor, M. R. (1994). *The search for meaning*. Nashville, TN: Abingdon Press.

Super, D. E. (1969). The natural history of a study of lives and vocations. *Perspectives on Education, 2*, 13–22.

Super, D. E. (1990). A life-span, life-space approach to career development. In D. Brown, L. Brooks & Associates, *Career choice and development: Applying contemporary theories to practice* (2nd ed.). San Francisco: Jossey-Bass.

Super, D. E. (1994). A life-span, life-space perspective on convergence. In M. L. Savikas & R. W. Lent (Eds.), *Convergence in career development theories*. Palo Alto, CA: Consulting Psychologists Press.

Yalom, I. D. (1980). *Existential therapy*. New York: Basic Books.

CHAPTER THREE

Work as Worth

Money or Meaning

Michael Demkovich
Dominican Ecclesial Institute

THE QUEST FOR self-knowledge brought the ancient
Greeks to the Pythia of Apollo. Her carved emblem, "know thyself," drew
people to this place of mystery. At Delphi, on the slopes of Mount
Parnassus, at the Earth's center, Greeks sought to divine life's meaning. In
cosmopolitan Athens, however, the Greeks turned to the goddess of wisdom, Athena, and these lovers of wisdom sought understanding. Delphi
now stand in ruins, but philosophy has reached far beyond Athens.

In this chapter, our quest for the self turns to the Athenian love of wisdom. Philosophy provides necessary tools for raising key metaphysical
questions in our search—questions about the nature of work, about society, and about the self. Plato and Aristotle, the premier Western philosophers, addressed these questions in light of society. In his *Republic,* Plato
sees society (and by extension work) as corresponding to the various
classes in a well-ordered state, a state wherein the most difficult labor
falls to those excluded from the state, the non-freeman. On the other hand,
Aristotle's *Politics* looks at society in light of the "household," both its running and its financing. These two thinkers set the stage for a philosophical
inquiry that needs to address work in relation to the nature of self and
society.

Though contemporary American culture is far removed from Athens, as
is most of Western culture, it is undeniably tethered to those categories
proper to philosophical questioning. The essence of this concept, the

nature of work, needs to be addressed so that the twentieth century can better understand the self in relation to work. After defining its nature, this chapter examines two approaches to understanding work. One approach views work in terms of its social and economic dimension, whereas the other sees it in terms of the person's moral and ethical becoming. With these two lenses, this chapter is able to raise important questions as to the present reality of the self, one's work, and one's relation to society.

WHAT IS WORK?

The question of self in work, at least as asked today, is clearly a post-Enlightenment concern; that is to say, it has its roots in the eighteenth century. Modernity's focus on the subject further qualifies the question by emphasizing the individual in a way that ancient philosophy did not. Consequently the nature of "work" must be understood from the perspective of the knowing subject, the ego, but it cannot ignore the larger social dimension.

Work, or labor, enters into the modern arena at roughly the same time that the American colonies declared their independence from England. It was the Scottish philosopher Adam Smith who shifted people's understanding of wealth away from an acquisition of gold and silver to a nation's ability to produce and acquire consumable goods. In *An Inquiry into the Nature and Cause of the Wealth of Nations,* Smith (1776/1981) calls for an economy that produces a surplus of the tradeable goods needed by the populace.[1] This in turn demands greater production and provides the base for exchanging goods. By a division of labor, productivity and workstations are increased. A person specializes in that form of production that covers his or her immediate needs and provides a surplus for trade or exchange.

For Smith, a person's pursuit of exchangeable goods contributed to the general welfare and resulted in an economy motivated by self-interest. It is capitalism that divides labor into individual laborers, producing and selling, so as to secure employment. Smith notes three aspects contributing to this division of labor that deserve particular attention in our quest for self. He states,

> This great increase of the quantity of work, which, in consequence of the division of labour, the same number of people are capable of performing, is owing

to three different circumstances; first, to the increase of dexterity in every particular workman; secondly, to the saving of the time which is commonly lost in passing from one species of work to another; and lastly, to the invention of a number of machines which facilitate and abridge labour, and enable one man to do the work of many. (Smith, 1776/1981, p. 17)

This division of labor meant a change in the understanding of work in three specific ways: (1) a specialization or particularization of the distinct operations in the process of production; (2) an increase in efficiency in the time required for the production of goods; and (3) a decrease in the number of workers due to the automation of some distinct operations.

Unlike preindustrial production methods, which required time for one person to complete all the steps by hand, this division of labor allowed a number of necessary workers to accomplish more in less time. Consequently, in light of the changes mentioned, work was seen as a particular part of the production, which employed fewer people aided by machines to produce more goods for sale in the same period of time it took one person to complete the entire process from beginning to end. The reason for this kind of labor was the production of a commodity that could be used to exchange for other commodities. As Smith observes, "Every man thus lives by exchanging, or becomes in some measure a merchant, and the society itself grows to be what is properly a commercial society" (1776/1981, p. 37).

Work, in the form of a wage, gives the worker the power to exchange goods according to their usefulness to the market. Differences among workers are similarly determined by their usefulness to the market. In defining the nature of work, this ability to engage ultimately in the exchange of goods so as to provide for one's life and well-being must be included. However, several aspects of work are hidden in Smith's division of labor corresponding to the three circumstances already mentioned. First, it seems that work now needs to be suited to the particular skills and talents of the worker (or the worker to the work), which raises problems as we experience labor's rapid development, its increasing technologies, and a constant resizing of its own divisions. Second, the new relation of work to time means that as work increases in efficient production, less time is required to produce goods useful to the market. Production now requires less work time, and theoretically workers enjoy more free time to be merchants exchanging in commercial society. This unexposed element of work is its implied consumerism. Finally, an overlooked aspect of work in commercial society is the constant elimination of old jobs and the introduction of new jobs demanded by efficiency, productivity, and automation.

One overlooked effect of this automation, or mechanization, which Berg (1988) examines, is the greater separation between home and workplace that machines created. This was especially damaging for women, who were confined to the home and family and consequently excluded from the public sphere of work. This distinction between the public and private spheres has implications for us when the mechanization, or more correctly home-computerization, is able to restore work to the home yet allow the home-worker, through this technology, access to the important social or public sphere. As old "jobs" are eliminated, new jobs and new places of work emerge. So whereas work gives a person economic power in society, every worker, even today, is beset by three variables: (1) the constant need to correlate one's skills to a specific job, and a job to one's skills; (2) the ambiguity involved in being both a producer and a consumer at the same time; and (3) the uncertainty about the continued usefulness of one's work to the market.

It is fair to say that *work* includes those actions that arise from self-interest and are done to acquire economic power in commercial society. In so defining work as acquiring economic power in commercial society, it is important to distinguish between those activities done for personal pleasure, such as sports, gardening, wood-working, and so on, and those same activities as work or a job, where they serve as a means to economic power in commercial society. We can add to this definition of work unpaid activities that contribute to one's economic power in commercial society, such as traditional housework, parenting, and volunteer work, which, although not a waged activity or hobby, do contribute to economic life. Benería (1988) has argued that conventional definitions of the labor force have "grossly underestimated" (p. 388) women's contributions. Her thesis can be extended to include all such nonwaged work and its implications for commercial society. Thus by definition work includes one's self-interest, the acquisition of economic power, and involvement in the public sphere of commercial society. Now we are able to turn our attention to specific approaches taken to locate work within social life.

APPROACHES OF
TWO DIFFERENT THINKERS

Karl Marx (1818–1883) first published his *Das Kapital* (in English, *Capital*) in 1867, almost a century after Adam Smith, and set out "to lay bare the economic law of motion of modern society" (Marx, p. 110); later, Maurice Blondel (1861–1939) treated the relation of thought to action in his 1893 work, *Action: Essay on a Critique of Life and a Science of Practice*.[2] It is impossible to cover the full breadth of these works, but it is possible to identify key insights as they apply to a philosophical understanding of work.

Karl Marx

In volume one of *Capital*, "The Process of Capitalist Production," one encounters some of the most difficult passages in Marx, for they are the most fundamental passages in understanding work, society, and self. One passage in particular offers a convenient capsule of Marx's thought:[3]

> [T]he labour of the individual asserts itself as a part of the labour of society, only by means of the relations which the act of exchange establishes directly between the products, and indirectly through them, between the producers. To the latter, therefore, the relations connecting the labour of one individual with that of the rest appear, not as direct social relations between individuals at work, but as they really are, material relations between persons and social relations between things. It is only by being exchanged that the products of labour acquire, as values, one uniform social status, distinct from their varied forms of existence as objects of utility. (Marx, 1887/1967, p. 73)

Marx's analysis sets out two critical realities: first, that the individual worker is an indirect part of the social economy; and second, that it is in the direct exchange of products that work or labor acquires value. Both of these realities imply the sense of self-alienation so present in Marx's earlier writing (*Economic and Philosophical Manuscripts,* 1844) and the constant subtext of *Capital*. The worker loses a sense of the social self as he or she alienates product and production into commodities. Work and self-worth are reduced to the monetary value of one's paycheck. It is obvious how easily income defines the self. The present necessity for two-income households is evident as the person is alienated from the self by a sense of monetary economic power: *I am what I own or am able to own*. Self-worth is seen in the exchange of money for goods (à la Adam Smith).

Marx's observations (although a complete study of his thought and its impact cannot be undertaken in this brief chapter) and his study of political economics had a major impact on late nineteenth-century communist society. His collaboration with Frederick Engels to establish the Communist party throughout Europe greatly altered the social order for the next century. The struggle of the worker to overthrow alienating class structures has served Marxist ideologies, with their emphasis on deterministic materialism, from the Soviet bloc to Latin American regimes. It is understandable that such a radical movement triggered various social, political, and philosophical reactions. Most notable among these reactions were existentialism and personalism, which in part characterized the early twentieth century's philosophical responses to Marxism (Kwant, 1960).

Maurice Blondel

There may be nothing more than historical coincidence that a decade after Marx's death in 1883 we find Maurice Blondel first publishing his controversial dissertation, *Action*. Whereas Marx presents work as self-alienating, Blondel sought to integrate human life from the perspective of experience and social action. Blondel's analysis of human action refocuses our question of the self and work away from work (as self-alienating) to self (as active agent). In *Action* (1893), Blondel presents the phenomenon of action in five critical stages that seem to move from subjective consciousness (stage one) to willed and intentional actions (stages two and three). This at last brings one from individual action to social and spiritual action (stages four and five). Unfortunately, Blondel speaks of this fifth stage as "superstitious action," which today implies an insignificance for true scholarship. On the contrary, what Blondel meant was human action directed toward subjugating the infinite, mysterious power.

It is in stage three that Blondel's analysis sheds special light on work and the self. By presenting a rather extensive inquiry into action, one far more metaphysical than Marx or Smith and much less a matter of economics, Blondel lays bare the intimate connection between human action and self-knowledge. Rather than treating action as solely volitional, he acknowledges the impact of one's actions on the actor: "There is then a perpetual circuit. Through voluntary operation we draw from ourselves power to move and to determine ourselves. . . . Through action, it seems that we get a grasp on ourselves from as far away as possible and that, underpinning the very foundations of our personal life, we move ourselves forward as a whole." (Blondel, 1883/1994, pp. 157–158)

By first understanding work as action, in Blondel's sense, we clearly see the self-constituting character of work and are able to ask questions about its ability to fashion and make the self. Blondel briefly touches on this as he treats the essential dimension of hard labor in understanding human action. He observes the human tendency to act in such labor:

> For all of us it is taxing to labor; no act of any impórtance reaches completion without some labor; and labor is passion in action, a suffering, an intimate contradiction. While I am concentrating my thought on the subject I am studying, I sense something like a spring that is trying to unwind, an attention ready to slip away, a bundle whose strands pull against the grasp of reflexion. Thus again, the members of the laborer, always subject to the same movements and compressed into the same mechanism, cry fatigue and pain. False and hateful, those slogans of a new morality, obviously meant to form to hard labor a people deprived of any higher encouragement: labor to hear these optimists, is alone agreeable, alone natural. No; to discipline our powers, a simple willing is not enough, nor even a single effort of our central energy; there has to be toil. Besides, labor has been looked on as a punishment, as an expiation, as ennobling for whoever has the courage to persevere in it freely without the constraint of need. And whatever may have been said, it is not the universal law in any degree, it is a properly human law. Only man does violence to himself, fights himself, makes himself suffer, kills himself, labors in acting. (Blondell, 1883/1994, pp. 158–159)

"Passion in action"[4] spends the self, and the repetition of movement brings about fatigue and pain. What is striking in Blondel's analysis is the moral character of this labor. The necessity of a moral motivation, be it punishment, restitution, or ennoblement, sets labor in a realm of action that is self-constituting and fundamentally social. "Passion in action" transforms the self. The agent, in acting, is acted upon, shaped and reshaped by the very doing. In light of our investigation, the self is constituted in action, in the work performed. This is why action or praxis can never be separate from moral and social action. Action (and work is included in this) constitutes the self, sometimes equal to the willed self, often unequal. The self is constituted not by what it knows or even by what it does but by what it becomes, actualizes in the doing. Work or labor then cannot be seen as merely monetary, a matter of money, but as part of the whole of human activity that constitutes the self, as a matter of meaning.

Action for Blondel is related to ultimate meaning and human destiny, which is integrative of self and society. He states,

> Man's need is to equal himself, so that nothing of what he is may remain alien or contrary to his willing, and nothing of what he wills may remain inaccessible or denied to his being. To act is to seek this agreement of knowing, willing and being, and to contribute in producing it or in compromising it. Action is the double movement which bears being to the end it is aiming at as to a new perfection, and which reintegrates the final cause into the efficient cause. (p. 425)

This agreement of knowing, willing, and being present in action (including labor) is crucial for self-integration of work and society.

Marx's and Blondel's Warning

Whereas Marx seems to ignore the self-constituting aspect (meaning) of work and human action,[5] Blondel seems unconcerned about the economic machinery of capitalism (money). However, both of these thinkers initiated a philosophical discussion on the worth of human existence that has continued to fuel the debate. Is the self alienated by modern society, with its division of labor and reduction of social relations to the exchange of commodities? Does a person really constitute the self by action independent of economic conditions, or better still, in spite of them? Is the worth of a person so tied to money that the moral character is abandoned? Or does self-worth depend on meaningful action no matter the pay or poverty? Capitalist and consumerist society definitely makes finding self-worth in work difficult. Blondel offers a wider scope in which to see work and self-worth, when labor is placed in the context of human action and human destiny. Our praxis (actions, trans-actions, labor, and so on) takes on a social character that undoes Marx's self-alienating exchange.

These philosophers highlight the difficulties of modern life with its need for economic autonomy, consumerist individualism, commercial society, and naive sense of human progress. Marx and Blondel anticipated our times, to warn us at the dawn of the third millennium that self, society, and work are the wealth and worth of the world. They critiqued the engine of modernity as it rolled off the assembly line, whereas the present age critiques postmodern society's alienation of self from action.

POSTMODERN SELF, WORK, AND SOCIETY

Thus far we have seen how the nature of society and work are intimately linked and that patterns in one affect the reality of the other. Adam Smith's "wealth of the nation" demanded a social order of commerce, and Karl Marx saw the consequences of this division of labor for the self as alienating worker from work. However, human existence is irrepressible, and Maurice Blondel offered up a philosophy of action that set work in the larger context of human action and human destiny, showing that self, society, and work are part of a mutually constitutive circuit. In other words, the self, in trans-acting (including work), constitutes the kind of society that dictates the kind of work valued by society. The kind of work valued by society in turn constitutes a dimension of the self (personally and socially).

The work of Kohn (1990) demonstrates the complex relations involved in the dimensions of work and personality often overlooked in social research on the subject of work. What is crucial in Blondel's analysis is his inclusion of that often overlooked moral character of all our human actions. Unfortunately, if the wealth or worth of a nation is seen in its economic commerce, the self, society, and work are reduced to a matter of increasing profits. Life is compartmentalized into a society divided according to private, public, and professional worlds, worlds that can exclude persons from fully integrating self, society, and work. The individual is so reduced to a matter of autonomy that "my job" is how I make "my money" and society exists for the protection of "my property," "my rights," and "my family."

Postmodernity, an often confusing notion, attempts to critique modernity from within the very limits of modernity itself. Its strongest criticism is aimed at subjectivity. Concurrent with this criticism, we find a suspicion about modernity's belief in metaphysical, historical, and psychological explanations that claim to answer all our questions. From a postmodern perspective, the quest for self in work is already an unfortunate formulation of the question, one defined by the ego and destined to the kind of idiosyncrasies already mentioned (my job, my salary, my property, and so forth). In a certain sense, Blondel anticipated the postmodern critique in emphasizing the *ethical character of human existence*. The criticism to be made of a Marxist understanding of labor is that capital economics attempts to offer too totalizing an answer, thus failing to do justice to the larger, more problematic realities.

This postmodern critique can be seen in sociology's own examination of the philosophical question of work, as seen in the 1990 collection of essays edited by Erikson and Vallas. In the final chapter, Vallas comments on the themes expressed by the twenty contributors to *The Nature of Work*, criticizing his fellow sociologists:[6]

> This lack of research on the relation between work and politics is not a random occurrence. Rather, it has a deeper source, stemming from [sociology's] failure to view work as part of a broader ensemble of social relations. Caught up in what Kanter has termed the "myth of separate worlds," occupational sociologists have long viewed the family as foreign to the study of work. We continue to view the community as the rightful province of urban sociologists, and so rarely inquire into the links between work and community (Kornblum, 1974). So too with the polity, with relations between dominant and minority groups, and so on. In all these cases, the structure of our own occupation impedes our grasp of the ways in which work is embedded in the wider social order. Increasingly, these divisions will need to be torn down. The development of the field requires that we transcend the divisions of intellectual labor we have ourselves devised. (p. 358)

This critique from sociology calls for the kind of interdisciplinary study of work to which the authors of this present volume are dedicated. Postmodern philosophy promotes a hermeneutics critical of the totalizing monolithic fields of academic specialization.

Emanuel Levinas (born 1906) is one of the original philosophers of the twentieth century whose writings (for example, *Justifications de l'ethique,* 1984) see ethics as the first philosophy. This Lithuanian-born Jew moved to Strasbourg in 1923 and later became a French citizen. During World War II, he was taken prisoner and placed in a Nazi labor camp (a perspective on labor unimagined by Marx or Blondel). Perhaps this is why Levinas's penetrating although brief treatment of work is so important. He places labor at a most peculiar place, at the point where self escapes the solitude of being. Postmodernity's critique of the modern self is that the self, left to the solitude of being, becomes self-absorbed. Levinas briefly discusses work in *Time and the Other,* but this one text captures for us the tone of his thought. He writes,

> The world offers the subject participation in existing in the form of enjoyment, and consequently permits it to exist at a distance from itself. The subject is absorbed in the object it absorbs, and nevertheless keeps a distance with regard

to that object. All enjoyment is also sensation—that is, knowledge and light. It is not just the disappearance of the self, but self-forgetfulness, as a first abnegation. (p. 67)

Labor or work frees the self from self-forgetfulness through the concrete reality of neediness. The necessity of work forces the self to grasp the nonself and in so doing discovers otherness, but it is a discovery born of pain and suffering. "In work—meaning, in effort, in its pain and sorrow—the subject finds the weight of the existence which involves its existent freedom itself. Pain and sorrow are the phenomena to which the solitude of the existent is finally reduced" (p. 68).

As fleeting as is Levinas's reference to work, it profoundly affects our quest for the self in work. Unlike the more enjoyable approach taken by Blondel, Levinas seems a hybrid of Marx and postmodernity. Work, precisely because of its kindredness with death via pain and sorrow, awakens the self (Marx might say alienates the self) from self-forgetfulness. Death confronts subjectivity with otherness that sets the self free from self-absorption so as to be "one-for-the-other."[7] Work, reduced to its pain and sorrow, forces the solitary self to leave its solitude and seek solidarity, to leave the autonomy of the ego and be for the other. Levinas, in *Time and the Other,* states, "Consequently only a being whose solitude has reached a crispation through suffering, and in relation with death, takes its place on a ground where the relationship with the other becomes possible" (p. 76).[8] Suffering, and here Levinas includes work, involuntarily compels the self, convulses the self into a social ground that allows one to relate with the other. Work, defined in this chapter as "action that arises from self-interest, done to acquire economic power in commercial society," now must mean that solidarity is of self-interest both personally and socially.

As strange as Levinas's thought appears to the modern thinker, he is not without profound application to our philosophical inquiry into self, society, and work. Rather than posing the problem from the perspective of a self that defines reality, Levinas begins with the assumption that the self is held hostage by its rational definitions, which reduce reality to a level of identity with the ego. The self, rather than being freed by self-understanding, is in fact locked into the solitude of ideologies. Unlike Marx's critique of work as self-alienating, Levinas sees this as forcefully freeing the self from self-absorption, self-forgetfulness. The division of labor that was so essential to Smith's wealth of the nation contained within its pain and suffering the liberation of self from solitude to solidarity with the other, the postmodern notion of alterity. Work, while the basis for economic life, is also the moral basis for social life. This is so, not in its capacity for commercial comfort but in its ethical demand to be for the other. Unemployment, or economic death, and our proximity to such pain, places the self on moral ground where it is possible to relate to the other socially and not commercially, for meaning, not money.

CONCLUSION

Although this chapter has sought a philosophical treatment of the self in work, it has only grazed the surface of Marx, Blondel, and Levinas as they assist our modern and postmodern inquiry. The quest for the self in work is a complex dynamic and is most satisfactorily addressed from the perspective of social solidarity and not the isolated self. Economic power, we have seen, ought not to be reduced to the alienating notion of wages or salary, because economic power is more social than monetary instruments.

In unemployment, the equivalent of economic death, we are forced from our self-absorption, our literal indebtedness to money, as we look to find new social relatedness (meaning to our life). Our capacity for human action confronts the self, now "out of sync" with social life and eager to redefine itself so as to reenter social relations. Familial systems intervene as the dislocated ego reassesses its relation to the public sphere, making "career" and "life" choices. This social network is made conscious of the kinds of work sanctioned by society and in turn reevaluates the kind of society promoted by such jobs.

The quest for the self in work is necessarily a quest for meaning, social relatedness. Although economic power is a significant means to achieving solidarity, it is not to be reduced to money as the basis for economic power. By examining the "broader ensemble of social relations" (Vallas, 1990), we discover the crucial link between work and community. While we are asking the question of the self in work, postmodernity is dislocating the self, forcing the question of work in community and community (solidarity) in the self. The pain and suffering that this entails, both personally and socially, frees us from our isolated self-absorption (Levinas, 1987). The quest for the self in work is by its nature simultaneously a quest for community. Plato and

Aristotle held this communal dimension and treated it under the notions of the state and the household (respectively). Even Marx hoped that the communal character of the workplace would shape communist society. Modernity's turn to the subject, the emergence of capitalism and consumerism in society, has forced the self into a definition too limited in terms of economic power. A philosophical framing of the question asks about the nature of self, work, and society, broadening the definition to include human action and social solidarity. Work as worth is much more a question of meaning than it is one about money. The worth of work is its critical appraisal, not only of the self's abilities to act and engage society in terms of economic power (utility) but also its sounding of the alarm on the limits in society itself (education, welfare, minimum wages, business, and so on) and the strains creating a new workplace (Kanter, 1990). What we do and why we do what we do as a society is the quest. What and whose actions are valued in the public sphere is the question. Are we willing to be changed through "passion in action?" (Blondel, 1893/1984, p. 158) This question is our work. Only in such a question do we approach the worth of work for the self.

NOTES

1. From *An Inquiry into the Nature and Cause of the Wealth of Nations,* by Adam Smith (W. B. Todd, Ed.), 1981 (Original work published 1776), Oxford, England: Oxford University Press. Reprinted with permission.

2. From *Action (1893): Essay on a Critique of Life and a Science of Practice,* by Maurice Blondel. Translated by Olivia Blanchette. ©1984 by the University of Notre Dame Press, Notre Dame, Indiana. Used by permission of the publisher.

3. From *Capital: A Critique of Political Economy,* Vol. 1 (p. 73), by Karl Marx (F. Engel, Ed., 3rd ed.) (S. Moore & E. Aveling, Trans.), 1967 (Original work published 1887), New York: International Publishers. Reprinted with permission.

4. The term *passion,* as used by Blondel, might be understood as strong emotion in action, but Blondel is using passion in the sense of *actio et passio.* Passion means the being acted upon as when we distinguish in grammar between the active and passive tense: "I threw the ball" (active); "The ball was thrown" (passive).

5. Later Marx places an expectation on the cooperative aspect of the factory workers, organized and relating to one another around a common task, as giving rise to a growing communist social awareness.

6. From Vallas, S. P. "Comments and Observations." In *The Nature of Work,* K. Erikson and S. P. Vallas (Eds.). ©1990 Yale University Press. Reprinted with permission.

7. See Levinas, E. (1981). *Otherwise Than Being or Beyond Essence* (A. Lingis, Trans.). The Hague: Martinus Nijhoff.

8. It needs to be noted that death for Levinas is in opposition to Heidegger's ontological sense of "being unto death." Earlier in *Time and the Other,* Levinas explains: "Death in Heidegger is an event of freedom, whereas for me the subject seems to reach the limit of the possible in suffering. It finds itself enchained, overwhelmed, and in some way passive. Death is in this sense the limit of idealism" (pp. 70–71).

REFERENCES

BBenería, L. (1988). Conceptualizing the labour force: The underestimation of women's economic activities. In R. E. Pahl (Ed.), *On work.* (pp. 372–391). Oxford, England: Basil Blackwell.

Berg, M. (1988). Women's work, mechanization, and the early phases of industrialization in England. In R. E. Pahl (Ed.), *On work* (pp. 61–94). Oxford, England: Basil Blackwell.

Blondel, M. (1984). *Action: Essay on a Critique of Life and a Science of Practice.* (O. Blanchette, Trans.). Notre Dame, IN: University of Notre Dame Press. (Original work published 1893)

Erikson, K., & Vallas, S. P. (Eds.). (1990). *The nature of work: Sociological perspectives.* New Haven, CT: Yale University Press.

Kanter, R. M. (1990). The new work force meets the changing workplace. In K. Erikson & S. P. Vallas (Eds.), *The nature of work* (pp. 279–303). New Haven, CT: Yale University Press.

Kohn, M. L. (1990). Unresolved issues in the relationship between work and personality. In K. Erikson & S. P. Vallas (Eds.), *The nature of work* (pp. 36–68). New Haven, CT: Yale University Press.

Kornblum, W. (1974). *Blue-collar community.* Chicago: University of Chicago Press.

Kwant, R. C. (1960). *Philosophy of labor.* Pittsburgh, PA: Duquesne University Press.

Levinas, E. (1981). *Otherwise than being or beyond essence* (A. Lingis, Trans.). The Hague: Martinus Nijhoff.

Levinas, E. (1984). *Justifications de l'éthique.* Bruxelles: Editiones de l'Université de Bruxelles.

Levinas, E. (1987). *Time and the other* (R. A. Cohen, Trans.). Pittsburgh, PA: Duquesne University Press.

Marx, K. (1967). *Capital: A critique of political economy* (Vols. 1–3). (F. Engel, Ed., 3rd ed.) (S. Moore & E. Aveling, Trans.). New York: International Publishers. (Original work published 1867)

Marx, K. (1967). *Economic and philosophical manuscripts of 1884.* Moscow: Progress Publishers.

Pahl, R. E. (Ed.). (1988). *On work: Historical, comparative, and theoretical approaches.* Oxford, England: Basil Blackwell.

Smith, A. (1981). *An inquiry into the nature and cause of the wealth of nations.* (Vols. 1–2). (R. H. Campbell, A. S. Skinner, & W. B. Todd, Eds.). Oxford, England: Oxford University Press. (Original work published 1776)

Vallas, S. P. (1990). Comments and observations. In K. Erikson & S. P. Vallas (Eds.), *The nature of work* (pp. 343–362). New Haven, CT: Yale University Press.

CHAPTER FOUR

Ready, Set, Grow

An Allegoric Induction into Quantum Careering

David V. Tiedeman
Lifecareer®[1] Foundation

THIS CHAPTER[2] IS partly inspired by the 1996 Summer Olympics in Atlanta, Georgia. Born in Americus, Georgia, I was duly impressed by the hospitality and conduct of my native state. Despite tragedy, the games transpired. Peace and joy seemed more prevalent than lawlessness and resentment, and the events made people of many nationalities feel a little closer.

Faced with choosing a metaphor for gently challenging excellence in personal existence in today's "medal-winning" perception of life as career (Miller-Tiedeman, 1988, 1989, 1992), I thought of the "ready, set, go" of sporting events.

READY

In 1962, Kuhn (1970) published *The Structure of Scientific Revolutions*. The book caused a stir in the scientific community. Breadth and depth of scholarship impressed, substance was novel but intriguing, and argument had the expected consistency. But scientists were not accustomed to thinking of nature's consistencies as *revolutionary*.

Over its thirty-five–year existence, Kuhn's book has influenced world society in many ways. It still graces the reference lists of many courses, both undergraduate and graduate, and is shelved in the "New Age" section in bookstores in major cities. As interest in paradigm shifts grows, Kuhn's scientific revolutions idea gains greater acceptance.

Kuhn's concept of "scientific revolution" provides context to our thesis here. Kuhn chose to use the histories of scientific advances big and powerful enough to have indelibly marked praxis worldwide to demonstrate that such changes are usually structural ones. The resulting models of such changes are called *paradigms*.

Two Relevant Scientific Revolutions

This chapter focuses on two career-relevant scientific revolutions occurring in the twentieth century: (1) the transition of Newtonian mechanics into quantum mechanics; and (2) a parallel transition of career mechanics into quantum career process (Miller-Tiedeman & Tiedeman, 1983; Miller-Tiedeman, 1988, 1989, 1992). These two transitions now coalesce. Personal transitioning from Newtonian to quantum mechanics serves as the necessary catalyst.

The transition from Newtonian to quantum mechanics started in a physical science that was older, further developed, and more disciplined than the career development field. However, career development grew up embedded in the Newtonian worldview, and its writings reflected that view until Miller-Tiedeman (1988) introduced the life-as-career theory which focused on the individual as theory maker. These two changes in theories will, beyond a reasonable doubt, affect the quality of life in the first half of the twenty-first century. After all, the ongoing transition from a Newtonian physics (Zukav, 1979) to a quantum physics fundamentally changes the very cosmos in which humans believe they live. Little wonder that such changes produce feelings of unfamiliarity, risk, anxiety, stress, and fear.

The paradigm shift from career mechanics to career process does not at present have the head of steam and import of the shift from Newtonian to quantum cosmos. However, signs indicate that a shift of that existential nature now waits in the wings of a universe theater ready to raise its curtain on a transition of the same order of magnitude.

The study of career as a science lives pretty close to the ground of its Newtonian roots to this day. This makes enlargement and diversification of career theory pretty tough. And that's tough on the growing demand for multiculturalism in the world. The human career is one area in which change toward multiculturalism is possible. Change can be achieved if citizens can master the process of self-counseling, which requires personal understanding of human consciousness *and* constructive use of that understanding. This bilevel activity (Koestler, 1964) requires familiarization and practice.

Introducing an Allegory

In this chapter, I will teach process while trying to empower process understanding. Children's writer A. A. Milne's (1926) characters, Pooh Bear and his friends, will help in allegorically connecting uninformed readers with quantum processes as they arise in our "virtual seminar." In a sense, this is like translating from English to French in a United Nations assembly meeting, where each delegate in need of translation receives such from his/her observer's booth upstairs. Here, Pooh Bear and his friends will offer you translation of quantum processes.

The author arrived allegorically and greeted his close friend Christopher Robin. "David, I'll give you a test," Christopher said. "Let's see how good you are at naming my Pooh friends after these many years from meeting them in Milne's books."

"OK, I'll take your dare," author David replied, "You, Christopher Robin, father to the forest creatures; Pooh Bear, your favorite, and source of wisdom through bumbling episodes; Eeyore, your gloomy and stubborn donkey; Owl, your wise old one; Piglet, one of your foils in adventuring; Kanga and her little Roo, your family with a lot of Kanga wisdom and Roo devilment; Tigger, your source of humor; and Rabbit, your speedster."

"You did fine. A. A. Milne seems to have had a good idea of names and events that would stick in memory," Christopher said. "Now why don't you give me a bit of background before tomorrow's seminar?"

Today's Career Underpinnings

"Christopher," David said, "traditional careerists tend to see their roots within the vocational context. But the scientific revolution on which today's career theory rests began with Nicolaus Copernicus, whose heliocentric view of cosmic rotation overthrew the geocentric view of Ptolemy and the Bible, which was the accepted dogma for more than a thousand years (Capra, 1982). René Descartes came along with his belief in the certainty of scientific knowledge. He even went so far as to conclude that nothing in the concept of body belongs to the mind and vice versa.

"Kepler derived laws of planetary motion and Galileo performed experiments to discover laws of falling bodies. Newton combined those two and formulated the general laws of motion for all macroscopic objects in the solar system. He believed these laws confirm the Cartesian view of nature.

"So in the late 1700s, Sir Isaac Newton's method of investigation became the accepted scientific method. His investigation of his hypotheses about the nature of gravity proved so successful that he captivated the scientific world for two centuries. We might even say Newton fired the mechanistic worldview shot heard round the world. This worldview persists even into our twentieth century.

"With a two-hundred–year backdrop of Newtonian physics, vocational guidance emerged in 1908 (Brewer, 1942). So in contrast to the revolution of Newtonian mechanics in the 1700s and 1800s, the vocational guidance revolution started from scratch in the 1900s. These two revolutions made deep inroads into human behavior and thought.

"In the early 1900s, the limits of Newtonian theory began appearing in atomic and subatomic experiments generally grouped as quantum mechanics (Capra, 1982). Reconciliation was needed, and a part of it was provided by Einstein's general theory of relativity ($e = mc^2$), where c is the speed of light. The Copenhagen Interpretation, conceived by twelve physicists of genius, provided a missing part of the needed transformation. *Abracadabra,* quantum mechanics *and* general relativity relegated Newtonian mechanics to a special-case theory. And the world literally changed in the perceptions of physicists, but few laypersons even seventy years later know the transformation or its important philosophical structure. Further, Zohar (1990) suggests that Newtonian physics is now considered so elementary that it's no longer taught at mainline universities."

SET

David continued to give Christopher background information. "Then what we today might call a quantum leap happened," he said. "In the beginning, instead of writing physics papers day after day, Capra (1975) started popularizing physics for the layperson. Soon Zukav (1979) popularized the space-time dimension of quantum mechanics, checking his understandings out with physicists. The popularity of these writings encouraged natural scientists in general to offer their views: Bohm (1980), Prigogine (1980), Swimme (1984), and more recently Hawking (1988, 1993). These books provide a solid core for a personal library on today's New Physics.

"This early splurge of books dovetailed with Miller-Tiedeman's discontent with career counseling assumptions and started her on the road to understanding what, if anything, the New Physics offered in parallels to life direction. It ended with her Lifecareer Theory (also known as quantum careering and living life as process) and philosophy (1983, 1988, 1989, 1992).

"As you make your developmental leap from a Newtonian to a quantum cosmology, never overlook your change from a supposedly stationary to a dynamic cosmos. The synergy (Fuller, 1981) of open collaboration during such growth, for the benefit of all, will point us to a greater appreciation of potential and value in life."

GROW

"Well, Christopher," said David, "as you might know, *grow* stands at the top of life's syllabus. Life keeps nudging its growth agenda forward in the universe, in individuals, in consciousness, and in social organizations (all this without a committee meeting)."

"You're right," said Christopher. "Maybe that's life's way of kicking humanity out of conformity. Which raises another question. Doesn't taking on a quantum mind-set unsettle your fifty-year career in Newtonian research?"

"You bet it unsettles me. But only in the sense that I wish I had known then what I know now," David said sadly. "So much to do, so little time. . .

"Read on and you'll see how I struggled with changing my paradigm, Christopher. I share this information because it may provide courage to those brave souls who dare to cross the Newtonian bridge to quantum understanding. At this point, it takes Karl Pribrim's notion of the *courage to look foolish* (Wilber, 1982) to support the start. If you don't invoke that stance, you discover you're learning more and more about less and less."

"OK, David," Christopher agreed amiably.

"I also share my paradigm change experience because it's part of the mandate in new paradigm research; that is, make clear where you are coming from in taking a particular view or espousing a particular idea, and, where appropriate, add experience to further explicate the idea (Reason & Rowan, 1981). You see in this approach, Christopher, the quantum notion that the cosmos is a web of relationships with space-time coordinates depends on where observer and object are placed. In other words, ideas birth out of more than reviews of literature.

Brief History

"But let's go on," said David. "Miller-Tiedeman has worked on this idea thirteen years. Even though we had numerous conversations, I only grasped the bottom line of the basic trust core of Erikson's (1959) psychosocial theory of identity formation when working to free myself from the Newtonian worldview. I then realized the importance of basic trust in any kind of personal change, particularly that of a worldview. I learned that too many differences exist between Newtonian and quantum theory to conceive of them as similar boxes fitting into one another from small to next larger to next larger and so on. But writing this chapter broke my reliance upon Newtonianism as the only paradigm for research.

"When I finally realized I simultaneously had to think revolutions in two theories, career and quantum," David began, "I opted for simplicity in attack. I therefore decided to visit Walden Pond, where Henry David Thoreau had in the nineteenth century so tellingly exemplified living attuned with nature, a core health outcome of today's Lifecareer theory/philosophy of going with, not against, the flow of life. Then I remembered that you, Pooh Bear, and the other Winnie-the-Pooh characters live no longer in England but at Walden Pond these days. That clinched my decision.

"Then I also recalled," David continued, "that your friends are very conscious of a need to adopt quantum careering as the universe continues to move evolutionarily forward on Prigogine's (1980) *arrow of time* into the ever more complex 'secrets' of the universe with which it teases and challenges humans to improve the quality of life on Earth" (Prigogine & Stengers, 1984).

At that point, Christopher suggested that he and David take a quick coffee break.

"A sterling idea, in my energy-depleted state," David replied as they walked into the kitchen to assess the coffee situation.

David and Christopher, with their coffee in hand, went back to their comfortable chairs in the living room.

Christopher asked David, "How did physics and career development come together? In a way they're unlikely bedfellows."

"Well, Christopher, in the late 1970s, at an ACA convention in Las Vegas, Miller-Tiedeman and I had dinner with Tom Kubistant and Dick Carhart. Somewhere in the conversation, Kubistant mentioned *The Dancing Wu Li Masters* (Zukav, 1979). This piqued Miller-Tiedeman's interest, and Kubistant said he would send her a copy. He did, and that marks day 1 in the birth of the quantum careering idea.

"In the spring of 1983, as president of the National Institute for the Advancement of Career Education headquartered at the University of Southern California, I had the opportunity to showcase the quantum process theory at an assembly to advance career. To support that quantum beginning, we invited Fritjof Capra (1983), physicist, as our keynote speaker.

"After the 1983 assembly, I worked with Miller-Tiedeman introducing Lifecareer to various groups. That experience led me to ask myself the following four questions: (1) What major characteristics do quantum and Lifecareer Theory both possess? (2) How do citizens and their counselors go about using the parallelism of quantum and career theories? (3) Can one individual really change the cosmic views of another? And (4) By what mechanism do new wholes manifest in dissipating self-organizing systems?

"With regard to my first quandary, both quantum and Lifecareer Theory are imbued with the same dynamic, universe energy, which is complementary to matter via $e=mc^2$. Complementary energy and matter grow and dance (Zukav, 1979). Hence quantum parallels include motion as primary, not holding on fearfully to what is now working while wondering what will happen when things change. Change happens each minute. And, as a specific energy configuration in universe energy, the Lifecareer Theory is but one example of quantum energy.

"With regard to my second quandary, you've got to shake the logical positivistic notion that a Newtonian paradigm is the only one worth considering. To do this, study process careering (Miller-Tiedeman, 1983, 1988, 1989, 1992), Reason & Rowan's (1981) new paradigm research ideas; Capra's (1975, 1982) New Physics ideas; Zukav's (1979) structure of quantum physics in nonmathematical terms; and Zohar's (1990) philosophy of quantum self.

"Also, talk with others about process career frequently. In living, writing about, or talking about process careering, notice how easily you can slip back into Newtonian thinking, as in changing careers, finding, or losing one. When you catch yourself falling back into that mind-set, you'll know you're on your way to changing your worldview. You'll also discover a new worldview doesn't spring full-blown like Minerva from Jupiter's forehead. It takes personal work. That separates those wanting quick fixes from those serious about change.

"With regard to my third quandary, it appeared that if I wanted to live the quantum process career (Lifecareer), I needed to start doing it. As my attitude toward process careering started to change, my worldview started to shift. That's why I subtitled this chapter 'An Allegorical Induction into Quantum Careering.' This chapter offers a virtual 'induction' to quantum careering, not just an 'introduction.' I had to change my own attitude before I could have any hope of facilitating change in another's attitude. This points up how important rhythm and timing are for each of us.

"My fourth quandary: My adopt-a-new-cosmos quandary lasted six months, during which I tried and revised theories, imposing them upon experience and revising over and over again. For instance, with my old Newtonian paradigm well intact, I went in to study for this seminar confident that I could derive new statistical techniques because I've done that (Rulon, Tiedeman, Tatsuoka, & Langmuir, 1967). I figured experienced me would grasp quantum theory in a jiffy. Nothing was farther from the truth. That's how a Newtonian framework fools you. *Present quantum theory for laypersons is not about changing formulas, it's about changing an attitude* (Capra, 1975). Quantum theory models the cosmos you must attitudinally assume to get the observations physicists are trying to boil down to the main ones.

"Christopher, attitudes don't change or gel readily. So don't expect yourself or your students to become quantumites overnight. But if you all stick with it, you'll find a new worldview."

"Why is a change of worldview difficult?" Christopher asked.

"Because it moves you into greater complexity. A self-organizing system always generates new wholes out of the chaos of dissipating structures (the Newtonian worldview). This is the order out of chaos often referred to by Prigogine and Stengers (1984). The dissipative structures idea won Prigogine the Nobel Prize in chemistry in 1977. It later became popularized as chaos theory.

"You know, Christopher," David continued, "self-organizing theory presumes that humans tend to grow into more differentiated and larger wholes both in the development of life phases and in their participation in the longer, slower evolutionary process in which their lives are also always participating. Like the universe as known to Prigogine (1980), we humans also tend toward more complexity even though sometimes we do it kicking and screaming as I did. But it's so much easier if you cooperate with the approaching forces while assessing the situation (Miller-Tiedeman, 1989).

"Now, what do you think of all this?"

Even the usually ebullient Christopher hesitated when asked for direct feedback. After a short pause, he bravely began. "You surely must have noted my interest. But quantum careering challenges the doubts, possible envies, and self-regards of leaders in career counseling. In addition, you bring those awakening to the precipices of unfamiliar change after teasing them with the hoards of figurative gold that exist in the creativity released in embracing quantum principles. You show them leaps are necessary. But you draw the mantle of physics around your ideas when you know full well that physics has been the course most readily avoided by college students, even yourself, for many years, as you tell me autobiographically."

"That's right, Christopher," David agreed. "It's true that I was not attracted to physics, to say nothing of linking it to career. But life works in interesting ways."

"It sure does," replied Christopher. "But I think I'm on overload now. So I'll just cooperate with the approaching force of sleep. See you tomorrow."

The Seminar Begins

The next morning, Christopher and David met Pooh walking to the seminar. Christopher introduced David and Pooh and asked Pooh if he would chair the seminar.

"It will be good experience for your university practicum," Christopher advised.

Christopher, David, and Pooh arrived at the seminar site together. Christopher made a quick survey, noting all Waldenites present and accounted for. He moved center stage, inviting David to come with him.

As was his habit before speaking, Christopher squared his shoulders and breathed a few deep abdominal breaths. "Friends," he said, "introductions are sufficient for us now to meet as old friends. But two dabs of additional orientation remain in order. I'm sure all of you appreciate Pooh's willingness to chair our seminar. In addition, Pooh told David and me that he had read all three Lifecareer books and heard University of Universe students discussing them. So, Pooh, please move to center stage now and share your knowledge and perspicacity."

Pooh rose and began. "Thank you, Christopher, for this chance to work with David, our distinguished guest. I'm in a student's dream role—teaching and learning virtually simultaneously. That's how time-sharing works in the big computer, isn't it, friends? It works fast in splitting several calls that are simultaneously feeding into the same territory. Electronic bits and pieces are transmitted and received without seeming interruption of any one of the computer's severally connected receivers' perceptions. I've been toying with that analogy lately as I try to understand what goes on in consciousness and process careering. But this seminar is yours to orient, not mine. So, David, I give you my friends, with confidence that a talker like me will find places to speak as we proceed."

Pooh, with a twinkle in his eye, took a figurative tricorn hat from behind his back and swept it toward David in a Yankee bow.

David moved center stage to the applause of his new friends. He too had a twinkle in his eye, acknowledging new friends who had mastered learning and personal development and looked forward to friendly discussion of some of the more important qualities of quantum careering.

Quantum Careering (Lifecareering) Along

David cleared his throat and began:

"I believe that to Lifecareer you need to check your worldview as frequently as you check the gas gauge of your car. Ask yourself, do you believe that the parts equal their whole or do you assert that the whole organizes the parts and is more than the sum of its parts? The former reflects Newtonian thinking; the latter quantum. If you don't get your worldviews sorted out like this, process living will elude you."

Rabbit, fast on the draw as usual, burst in and excitedly asked, "What does a worldview have to do with anything?"

"Well," David replied calmly, "your worldview reflects your beliefs and values, which influence your decisions. So a worldview anchors your actions and behavior. Historically the emphasis has been and still is on identifying skills, abilities, and interests, then getting occupational information in order to match yourself to the right job. Career is considered something you search for, lose, find, and go on to find a second, third, and fourth time. You see, Rabbit, career theory has been pretty much an outside job. Traditionalists have tended to dumb down clients, not smarten them up.

"Supporting intelligence means accepting personal knowledge as the primary and best occupational information. On the other hand, you recognize that the individual's intelligence will prompt him or her to gather any external secondary information needed. This approach indicates that you understand how personal data for each of us changes moment by moment as experience changes. That's why you need to check your worldview often, using the question, Am I living process using my personal theory, or am I hung up in the old Newtonian worldview following traditional thinking that doesn't acknowledge me as a theory maker? It's amazing how easily you can slip back into that old view without even noticing it."

Discussion

David then restated his thesis: "Two important career-relevant revolutions occurred during the twentieth century—quantum mechanics began replacing Newtonian mechanics in subatomic realms, and process-career theory started displacing occupational selection in adolescent years. Quantum mechanics and Einstein's provision of his general theory of relativity, $e=mc^2$, linked both of these revolutions.

"Concerning quantum theory, twelve outstanding physicists met in Brussels in the summer of 1924 and agreed that quantum theory is about correlations in our experience. They further said, 'It doesn't matter what quantum mechanics is about. The important thing is that it works' (Zukav, 1979, p. 62). These statements became known as the Copenhagen Interpretation. Zukav calls this acceptance "one of the most important statements in the history of science" (p. 62). The rational part of our psyche began to merge again with our nonbelieving side. About thirty years later, physicists joined Einstein's general theory of relativity with quantum mechanics. They called this a *scatter* or *s-matrix*. The s-matrix enabled physicists to reproduce quite accurately the paths into which several kinds of high-energy particles scattered upon encountering other high-energy particles.

"Concerning quantum careering: In 1983, Anna Miller-Tiedeman introduced quantum careering to the career development field and it became known as the Lifecareer Theory. This led the first attempt to integrate quantum physics and career, which introduced the individual as theory maker. This effort of responsible self-direction needs encouragement as the crossover to quantum thinking will in most instances produce pain. But the elimination of the old handcuffs of Newtonian thought will bring new awareness and freedom."

"But David," Kanga hesitantly joined in, "quantum mechanics doesn't replace Newtonian mechanics, does it?"

"The answer is simply that quantum mechanics subordinates Newtonian mechanics as a special-case theory. But in circumstances where Newtonian Theory works, it's stunning, like getting us on the moon."

"David, it sounds to me like we need to help each other grow into quantum understanding because it's not easy and support can ease the way," said Pooh. "As I remember the accommodation step in your decision-making paradigm (Tiedeman, 1963), the first stage would be *induction,* where the idea gets tested knowing there's a lot to learn. When the individual starts to feel comfortable with quantum, this brings on the *reformation phase,* in which the reformer believes everyone should move in a certain direction. But after some meaningful personal experiences provide an actionable base, the reformer moves into *reintegration,* realizing that everyone moves at his or her own rate of understanding, which is constitutionally guaranteed to American citizens."

Rabbit quickly added, "Crossing the bridge to quantum takes a lot of trust, perhaps way beyond Erikson's (1959) basic trust. But even more difficult is holding that trust, particularly when the majority isn't supporting it. This certainly makes it the 'road less traveled,' doesn't it?"

"That's true," replied David, "but we need to recognize, as Prigogine (1980) demonstrates, that life always moves into greater complexity. None of us have a choice about that. Our only choice is, do we try to understand the new and cooperate with it or do we remain in the backwaters?"

Kanga said, "I suppose quantum process refers to some of the presumed actions of electrons when physicists put an electron source into a linear accelerator and bombard the receptor with another electron source. As I understand it, under those conditions, physicists excite atoms so much that they eventually 'leap' out of the nucleus ring in which they rotate when unexcited."

"Isn't that what the TV show *Quantum Leap* does when the space travel-er drops in and out of time zones?" Rabbit demanded a little petulantly, because not responding first, as well as fearing loss of face, if wrong, embarrassed him. Notice the process veered from different meanings of process to Rabbit's need to jump into quantum process, a specific kind of process. That's a quantum characteristic.

"Yes, Rabbit," David said consolingly, a bit more conscious of what costs people pay for public participation in learning "process." "But I didn't expect to get that illustration of process so soon in the seminar.

"While we're on the point, Rabbit, it's a good time to suggest recogniz-ing quantum mechanics roots from two theories. One root will be the elec-tron and subatomic phenomena of what is commonly called 'quantum the-ory.' The other root of quantum mechanics will be relativity theory. The resulting s-matrix is the way scientists build, from stepping stone to step-ping stone."

A young voice came from the other end of the seminar room. "I know what relativity theory is," the voice said, "$e = mc^2$. Energy equals the prod-uct of mass times the square of c, the speed of light. Energy and mass are complementary. You can convert energy to mass and mass to energy."

"Wait a minute," David said, trying to contain his surprise at the inten-sity of the voice and its owner's possession of so many facts of relativity the-ory. "Who are you? With all your knowledge of relativity, you might tutor Christopher's friends who want to learn more about the concepts we'll just skim in this seminar."

"That would be fun," the little voice replied. "I'm Roo, son of Kanga who sits beside me. Christopher sent me to public school, where they taught me a lot about the atomic and subatomic worlds."

Because Roo brought it up, David then offered short sound bites about relativity a little earlier than he had planned. That's another characteristic of process: It dictates the content, but, interestingly, all gets covered, although not in what we ordinarily call logical order—process doesn't always cooperate with logic. That tends to frustrate us; that's when we sometimes break the flow to try to bend it back to logic. That's when we slip back down the slope of the Newtonian worldview.

Roo then asked, "Why can't we stop ourselves?"

David replied, "Because we're so used to doing it. It's what we call habit. And you know how hard habit is to break.

"As I understand it," David continued, "space and time are not independent; they exist as the four dimensions: the conventional three dimensions of space—length, width, and depth—and time as the fourth dimension in space-time curves. The potential curving of space in the four space-time dimensions may even be the result of present incapacity in most human consciousness to experience these projections from a five-dimensional space-time and 'suchness' spirit matrix. 'Suchness' can't be seen; it must be inferred. Inference is easy in matrix algebra—simply add another column to the matrix already representing four-dimensional data. Essentially this gives you the advantage of inferring capacity to 'see' the ball of the usual three dimensions moving through time as our spaceships do in any cartoonist's representation of Earth rotating directionally through the space-time matrix. The fifth dimension is then inferred as something like a cut-in of a spaceship's engines to overcome the effects of time compression as the spaceship nears infinity. That's the physical reference to the dimension of suchness.

Fifth dimensions are available to behavioral scientists as the fifth canonical root of their principal components analyses.

"Further human movement into subtle, causal, and spiritual realms in consciousness seems to hinge on moving consciousness first into the space-time or subtlety-consciousness dimension of Einstein's theory of relativity and then beyond into suchness spirit—the fifth and sixth dimensions, which bring understanding of the causal and spiritual dimensions of consciousness. In this regard, Eastern mysticism seems to have already advanced human beings into such states of consciousness, which are not commonly realized in our Western culture" (Capra, 1975, 1982).

David then complimented Christopher's friends: "Since you all seem pretty well oriented to quantum theory as a whole, I have no intention of providing an elementary text on atomic physics. I will, however, with your concurrence, introduce quantum physics concepts because they offer compelling parallels we can learn from to better understand our own approach and thinking."

"David," Christopher requested, "before you introduce those principles, please tell us a little about how this quantum thing came about."

"I'd like to tackle that," Wise Old Owl chimed in. David, glad to see seminar interest spreading, nodded and smiled.

Owl, following his usual "hhrumph," said, "Scientists and nature got along pretty cooperatively in developing scientific understanding from the

Renaissance to the twentieth century. Nature had given physical scientists a number of yes answers to their theory-guided inquiries about levers, inclined planes, pendulums, light, sound, heat, magnetism, gravity, and the like. Various constants and several important ratios had been unified by using field concepts. Nature knows her logic with demonstrably little variation in results among individuals who take care to do exactly as directed by the discoverer of those seeming constants of nature.

"As several of these fundamental constants and ratios were identified and satisfactorily stabilized, a new era of scientific activities set in—higher level cognitive skills such as comparison, noting distinctions, attributing and verifying differences when possible. These, of course, are elements of generalization. To humans, then, mind seems built on consciousness 'blocks' such as (1) data, idea, trial; (2) data, idea, trial at a higher level, and so on. This is one procedure that mind uses in coming to understanding. Nature participates in such constructionist communications with humans. However, nature is in no hurry to volunteer information. Humans therefore have to work for it, experiment, that is," continued Owl, the forest's philosopher of science.

At this point, trickster Tigger pounced into the discussion. "But as you might guess," Tigger offered, "former centuries have not all been years of milk and honey for humans who elect, as Buckminster Fuller did (1981), to pattern their lives on what they themselves come to know experientially, not on what they have been ordered to do. But truth strongly appeals to some humans despite the obstacles other humans erect to slow the sharing of advances throughout the universe.

"So New Physics emerged as the world turned steadily. Physical science had already dropped several soul-disturbing changes of view on the good burghers of Europe by the end of the Renaissance. For instance, it had been determined that Earth rotated about our sun, not the sun around the Earth. When Columbus wanted to make his expeditions to the New World, the masses cried, 'The world is flat and he'll fall off.' As we all know today, he didn't fall off, nor did he discover a New World. The 'West Indians' were already here. Today those changes in conventional cosmological grounds seem almost inconsequential. But they don't seem so tranquil to people experiencing them while they happen. Existential change is no bed of roses.

"In continuing to discover principle upon principle, specific by specific, physicists began to unfold the secrets of extant results, which later revealed themselves as parts of a more general phenomenon. This is another illustration of life moving toward more complexity as Prigogine (1980) contends. Life just won't stand still. It loves to grow, irrespective of our inclinations that way. And the New Physics is but one in an infinity of examples of how life continues to do that. The quantum and career process in consciousness union marks another example."

Kanga joined the discussion of quantum processes. "I've been listening carefully," she started. "I've an intuition about unity. I'm probably wide of the mark, but the quantum process tolerates less than certainty, right?"

"A whole lot less than certainty. In fact, it's all uncertainty," replied David. "In shifting from an elemental to a quantum-relativistic view of mechanics and energy in the universe, physicists had to move from only attending to elements to more inclusive attention to relationships in self-managed systems in general. And importantly, the quantum paradigm includes experiential approximations, while Newtonian mechanics doesn't" (Capra, 1982).

Pooh asked quizzically, "If physicists use experiential approximations, why don't we do the same about career? After all, career is but another universe-complementary manifestation of energy and therefore subject to all universe concepts."

"Even though quantum physics was discovered in the 1900s, it has not penetrated deeply into many disciplines, not even career development," replied David. "In addition, there's something to Kuhn's (1970) notion that paradigms don't usually change at the top. They start at the edges and go in or at the bottom and go up as those at the top seem too vested in the old.

"You might think of it as Heifetz does in his book *Leadership Without Easy Answers* (1994). He maintains that good leadership means going to the balcony periodically and observing the action on the dance floor below. In that sense, Miller-Tiedeman did just that. She stepped to the career development balcony and started asking questions from the quantum viewpoint.

"She was aided by her deep understanding that life's career is renewal, along with several other factors: (1) She reads from the collective intelligence (that's another story) and places great confidence in it; (2) she learned from her experience; and (3) she listened to her inner wisdom and acted on the larger theoretical framework toward which life pulled her. So she didn't decide to write a process theory—it evolved in her experience. That's an important process understanding.

"Probably as important, she took the physics attitude she learned when Capra (1983) keynoted a 1983 assembly to advance career. Capra suggested that physicists take a pragmatic attitude about any approach. When they have a certain theory that they think isn't quite sound, mathematically or otherwise, but it works, then they say, 'Well, there must be something to it.' They then use the theory and work out the details later."

"Before we move on," Pooh suggested, "let me note how the process of ideas jumping from mind to mind again takes us over and encourages us to probe deeper. That's intelligence at work in consciousness. It doesn't abide by rules; it just keeps tumbling around and around like crystals in a kaleidoscope making new patterns time after time after time. It rather resembles what the electrons, photons, mesons, and nucleons do. 'They lead double lives as they are: now position; now momentum; now particles; now waves; now mass; now energy-all in response to each other and to the environment'" (Zohar, 1990, p. 98).

Eeyore sensed the rising tide of understanding in the seminar and willingly stopped being a stubborn Newtonian to contribute his growing understanding of quantum mechanics.

"Quantum mechanics forms a dynamic whole," he said. "Quantum wholes are always greater than the sum of their parts. This is true in metal alloys and it's also true for groups. We're more together than we are apart. Only by putting the parts of a former whole into what may look like a virtual whole as in a completed jigsaw puzzle can you restore the pieces of a supposed whole into the semblance of a true whole. This is an important and difficult conceptual/perceptual change for any who will switch from the Newtonian paradigm to the quantum one. You must speak actively and tentatively in quantum if it is to work. But you're taught to speak passively and with certainty in the Newtonian framework if you want to do things right, forgetting about the higher level of doing right things creatively.

"Attitudes of a few about the nature of consciousness and the universe shifted as physicists attempted to gain more fundamental understanding of what their mathematics told them was necessary for more adequate correspondence between their models and their observations. The search for more fundamental concepts persisted in physics in marked contrast to the habits we Newtonian career psychologists and counselors ordinarily exhibit of accepting the empirical with little or no thought into more far-reaching principles that reveal understanding, not mere satisfaction."

PRINCIPLES TO GROW ON

"I'll briefly review the following physics principles introduced to the career development field in 1983 and in subsequent publications (Miller-Tiedeman, 1983, 1988, 1989, 1992)," said David. "You may find them useful as you teach your University of Universe students about quantum careering. That way you help these principles into more active use in our now so empirically defined, Newtonian-based career psychology."

Principle 1. The uncertainty principle. "The more you concentrate on the measurement of one thing, the less you know of another in complement with it," explained David. "For instance, the more you know of elements, the less you know of their momentum and vice versa. When you consider parallels to this idea, you also see this principle in all of life. For instance, when you advise a client, you introduce major uncertainty. Why? Because you have no way of guaranteeing any outcome because the next minute both you and the client change. Career counseling is all conjecture with a multiplicity of possibilities, many of which may not have come up in a session."

Rabbit piped up: "But from what I've been hearing, there are also quantum certainties, like change, movement, and even uncertainty. It's just that we have to retune our worldviews, as you said earlier. I also find I feel better physically when I don't depend on anything. I then start to wonder why people didn't notice this before. But I suppose it all takes time."

Piglet added, "I know what you mean. My study suggests that when you count on something to happen and it doesn't, you tend to feel stressed, and stress kills off immune cells (Miller-Tiedeman, 1996). Yes, I find the link between life direction and stress powerful in terms of becoming aware and potentially changing our behavior."

Kanga started to catch on to process and noted again how group members veered away from the main information by offering their own intelligence. "That's the way we'll all start to understand quantum. We have to tell our individual stories that illustrate the concept. While no one else can duplicate my story, it always helps to hear someone else's perspective. OK, go on, David."

Principle 2. In logical positivistic psychology, error is a basic concept. "Measures are picked or constructed to minimize error," David went on. "In quantum mechanics, error is the seeming nuisance we tolerate because we cannot predict with 100 percent accuracy. The uncertainty principle awakens us to the fact that we are never going to predict with 100 percent accuracy. We cannot know everything. We cannot guide to any ultimate truth for another. In addition, psychometrics delineated by maximizing individual differences as in logical positivism may separate individuals from individuals as can best be done. But if it will not tell us anything about the individual's life journey and vice versa, you need intrapersonal data for that purpose."

Rabbit said, "Then the research will need to change, won't it?"

"Yes. Just notice the language of research—dependent and independent variables. This assumes people can be reduced to a set of variables across persons and situations. When you elevate the individual to theory maker, those assumptions won't work. But the process remains the same. Reason and Rowan (1981) suggest that new paradigm research is a systematic approach to inquiry, a rigorous search for truth, which does not kill off all it touches. This new approach can be seen as a synthesis of naive inquiry and orthodox research.

"Another aspect of new paradigm research is making clear where one is coming from in taking a particular view. 'That's what I did in sharing a brief history of both science and quantum careering. Traditionally that is done by references to previous work. But Reason and Rowan (1981) think it important to politics, current work and relationships, general way of being in the world, or whatever. They suggest that acknowledging intellectual debt ought to go back even to ancient times, not just the last five years, which is usually the case in academia. In literature review, new paradigm research would work across disciplines, looking at works of philosophy, theology, history, literature, and multidisciplinary searches with the social science. We ought to watch that we don't fall in love with our numerics so much that they are precise but not true. Statistical significance may have no human use and it may be that it's better to be deeply interesting than accurately boring."

Principle 3. Complementarity. "If you change one thing in a system, other things change throughout the system. A system is of a whole. Additionally, when you focus on one thing you miss others.

"For instance, hundreds of students enter counseling and psychology programs each semester hoping to work in private practice or a health-related organization. They evidently believe they're training for something that will support them. However, if you look on the other side—managed care, HMOs, and insurance companies—you find that talk therapy now gives way to drug therapy. For instance, some insurance companies allow four therapy sessions, and then it's on to drug therapy. Critser (1996), in his essay, "Oh How Happy We'll Be," said that in the late 1980s, of the nearly sixteen million patients who visited doctors for depression, seventy percent ended up in drug therapy (p. 44). Drug therapy is not coming, it's here big time. If an individual wanted to be on the upside of the wave, he or she might consider training as a pharmacologist. When you focus on any discipline without looking at the totality of which that discipline is only a part, you miss other possibilities, one of which may be a lower income."

Principle 4. The whole is more than the sum of its parts. "The whole is in each of its parts, but the whole cannot be reconstructed from its parts," said David. "This synergistic quantum principle of growth stands in contrast to the Boltzmann second law of thermodynamics, which suggests that energy tends toward decay or entropy without overall growth.

"Technologically, humans first experienced synergy in the 1860s, when world navies began using metal alloys in ship construction because the tensile strengths of alloys are greater than the sum of tensile strengths of their pure metal parts.

"In career psychology, we presently bury this wholeness phenomenon in the errors of our models of individual differences with which we presently guide the careers of our students. We can never escape from the self-renewing functions of self-organizing systems into their self-transcending functions until we and our learners take our sense of living wholes into consideration in our systems of individual thought and action."

Principle 5. The observer cannot separate him- or herself from what she or he observes. "We find what we look for," David went on. "This principle appears in each of our observations. If we look for elements in matter, we find them; if we look for quanta in matter, we find them.

"We needlessly attempt to rid our instruments of ourselves. But we actually do our best in measuring when we not only read ourselves into our measurements but also share responsibility for the measurement process and results with our learners, who have the ultimate responsibility for what they now know, think, and find.

"On an everyday level, you can see this principle frequently when you look for something and because it's not in the shape or package you remembered, you fail to see it. If it's something that doesn't interest you, you don't see it. Taking that into the paradigm area, if you don't believe something, you don't see it.

"If you'll remember, the Swiss invented the quartz watch but missed the market because they didn't believe it would replace the watch with bearings (Barker, 1990). The same thing happened when several large companies missed the Xerox invention."

Principle 6. Interrelationship, interconnection, and interpenetration are the rules, not the exception. "Contrary to Western cultural notions, independence does not exist in the universe, rugged individualism notwithstanding. Wholeness perpetually works in the universe. Conceptual consciousness works in the balance of particulars and wholes, which we humans experience as paradox."

Principle 7. Nonlocal connections. "In the subatomic realm, changing the spin of a particle in Vancouver simultaneously counterrotates a particle in Montreal, speaking figuratively, that is," said David. "Interestingly, the nonlocal connection seems to operate at a speed exceeding that of light.

"In career, we keep looking at what is. But every *what is* exists with a *what is not*. Furthermore, *what is not* ordinarily possesses more powerful energies than *what is*. Hence if we and our learners follow evolutionary movement of life consciousness into general-purpose quantum being, we must learn to deal with both the *what is* and *what is not* in every cognitive experience and to tune in perceptually on the holistically operating life consciousness in each of us (Prigogine, 1980). Our intuitions are the nonlocal connections with incisive detail, at work in our attentive consciousness. We give these nonlocal intuitive connections the opportunity to guide our attentive consciousness by opening our attention, perhaps meditatively, to more comprehensive consciousness."

Pooh, with a worried look, said, "This whole business of process scares me. I worry that we'll each start growing in different ways and directions and everything will fall apart."

Owl hurriedly replied, "Pooh, you're forgetting about self-organizing systems. We may fall apart and decide our current group isn't for us. But then we turn around and surprisingly find a new group very friendly to our ideas. It seems we get tunnel vision thinking that the group we're in is the only group and nothing else exists. That's just where humanity currently stands in its evolution. But enough people now break out and find new groups and that courages the rest of us."

Pooh asked, "Why did you make *courage* a verb?"

Owl replied, "Because when you start thinking motion and movement, many nouns can metamorphose into verbs. Bohm (1980) has a chapter on the need for a new language. This will buzz grammarians, but even they can't escape progress."

"That's right," replied David. "But let's look back now and notice how life has reorganized over the last hundred years."

TOWARD REINTEGRATION

Ready: A Look Back

"The quest for accuracy, flexibility, speed, wholeness, and greater complexity in human/nature interactions intensified in the twentieth century," explained David. "Increasing attention to science was at the core of that intensification. Humans had already somewhat accelerated their learning of science and nature interactions. More and more details had been added to human understanding of various natural and humanly implicated conditions of nature and humanity. More slowly, but still accelerating, nature and humans had also learned to converse at a more general level, one in which more detail was being accommodated with increasingly less complicated but more powerful mathematical shorthand for humans to understand.

"In the twentieth century, humans brought science out of musty academic closets into the public domain. Now, by century's end, science seems as much at home in radio and TV talk shows, educational programs, and entertainment as it is in schools and colleges. Politicians and commentators delight in telling who is leading whom in what kind of 'scientific poll.' Probability, DNA, and the impossibility of anything being known with certainty figured mightily in the life-or-death trial of an accused murderer.

"Economics, psychology, and counseling get so specialized that citizens frequently can't cope for not knowing which pea of truth is under which of several thousand walnut shells the gods of chance shuffle under our noses. Fortunately nature's self-correcting properties save those who like to gamble. 'Ante-up or quit' begins flashing in their minds, warning that more than money is now at stake: There are matters such as reputation, foolish use of credit, even death. Finally, some realize it's a losing game if they are playing against a large bank and play is of sufficiently long duration for the bank to win on size and endurance."

Set: In Progress

"In a similar vein, the 'bean counters' of banking are quietly but openly putting money out of circulation. Credit cards are now being rather generously distributed. They will become the coin of the realm.

"America will downsize from Galbraith's affluent society into what I foresee a 'Junior Galbraith' may write: *The New America: The Credit Society*. Banks and government will happily grant you ever more credit if they can profit from doing so. Banks and governments will know how each of us stands. Don't expect to know that yourself. Sure, banks and governments will reveal where you stand whenever asked. But neither you nor banks nor governments can adjust your account balances for the time lapse between their last entry and your last expenditure or payment request. That's the complementarity principle. You don't know or care what system the accountants use, and they don't know what you have done in the last millionth of a second when you made your last electronic transfer to your Swiss bank account. (That's the uncertainty principle.)

"You don't have to tease yourself long and arduously with the discourse of these risks humans and nature accept before you undermine your confidence. So let's return to understanding how humans and nature learn to converse and cooperate."

Grow: In Quantum Careering

"The key to moving forward in life, whether in a job or in general, is found by a cooperative relationship with life. The key to that improvement will be found in support of individuals' unfoldments toward ever more perfect manifestations of themselves as atomic energy rather than as atomic particles (Bohm, 1980). This seems to be the present conventional thinking of physicists. Energy is the most basic force in the universe. Einstein's simple relationship between energy and particles, namely $e = mc^2$, where c equals the speed of light, governs the transformation of energy from one manifestation to the other and back. The relationship is complementary, reciprocating.

"The change process inheres in the reciprocating relationship of energy and particles. That change process functions as a self-organizing system. Give yourself to that change process with understanding and you will not only begin to know self-organizing systems in general, but you will also discern new means of understanding consciousness and spirit.

"This has been an exciting seminar," concluded David. "So many possible futures. I express deep gratitude to every one of you new friends. Your interest and thought impress me. I can well see how you and Christopher get on so well. You have become a multicultural family demonstrating friendship among cultures at all times. Such love and support will bring us peacefully through some of the many troublesome spots in today's world."

David admitted to himself that the road had been long and tiring and uncertainty a constant companion while his new learning was becoming familiar. God must have loved ambiguity since he created so much of it, he thought with a chuckle. But that's the oil in the wheel of life.

CONCLUSION

At this juncture in my own quantum career, I join my faith with Miller-Tiedeman and with Lee Richmond, who has worked with us for a decade to leave to posterity what we believe has endless life for those daring to appreciate the 99 percent invisible in the universe (Fuller, 1981).

May these good Irish wishes accompany you on your personal journey to spirit in life:

> As you walk courageously into your own quantum experience:
> May the road rise up to meet you as you consider yourself a theory maker.
> May the wind always be at your back as you reach for higher understanding.
> May the sun shine warm upon your face when you need support.
> May the rains fall soft upon your fields when you need nourishment.
> And until we meet again, may God hold you in his all-encompassing quantum consciousness—today's ultimate state of oneness.
> (adapted from an old Irish poem)

NOTES

1. Lifecareer and Life-Is-Career are registered trademarks of the Lifecareer Foundation.

2. I acknowledge my debt to Anna Miller-Tiedeman, her tenacity of belief in process and long-term thought about quantum careering, which she freely shared in advising and assessing me in this writing. I am honored to be her colleague in showing that love and truth can coexist as they must for spirit to come alive in work.

REFERENCES

Barker, J. A. (1990). The business of paradigms: Discovering the future [Video]. Burnsvine, MN: Charthouse International Learning Corporation.

Bohm, D. (1980). *Wholeness and the implicate order.* New York: Routledge.

Brewer, J. M. (1942). *History of vocational guidance: Origins and early development.* New York: HarperCollins.

Capra, F. (1975). *The tao of physics.* Boston: Shambhala.

Capra, F. (1982). *The turning point: Science, society, and the rising culture.* New York: Simon & Schuster.

Capra, F. (1983). The turning point. In C. Lynch, A. Miller-Tiedeman, & D. V. Tiedeman (Eds.), *Proceedings of the 1983 Assembly to Advance Career.* Vista, CA: Lifecareer® Foundation.

Critser, G. (1996, June). Oh how happy we'll be. *Harper's,* 39–48.

Erikson, E. H. (1959). Identity and the life cycle: Selected papers. In *Psychological Issues,* Vol. 1, Essay 1. New York: International Universities Press.

Feller, R., & Walz, G. (Eds.). (1996). *Career transitions in turbulent times.* Greensboro, NC: ERIC/CASS Publications.

Fuller, B. (1981). *Critical path.* New York: St. Martin's Press.

Hawking, S. (1988). *A brief history of time: From the big bang to black holes.* New York: Bantam Books.

Hawking, S. (1993). *Black holes and baby universes and other essays.* New York: Bantam Books.

Heifetz, R. (1994). *Leadership without easy answers.* Cambridge, MA: Belknap Press.

Koestler, A. (1964). *The act of creation: A study of the conscious and unconscious in science and art.* New York: Dell.

Kuhn, T. S. (1970). *The structure of scientific revolutions.* Chicago: University of Chicago Press.

Miller-Tiedeman, A. (1988). *LIFECAREER: The quantum leap into a process theory of career.* Vista, CA: Lifecareer® Foundation.

Miller-Tiedeman, A. (1989). *How NOT to make it . . . and succeed: The truth about your Lifecareer.* Vista, CA: Lifecareer® Foundation.

Miller-Tiedeman, A. (1992). *LIFECAREER: How it can benefit you.* Vista, CA: Lifecareer® Foundation.

Miller-Tiedeman, A. (1996). Surfing the quantum: Notes of a Lifecareer® developing. In R. Feller & G. Walz (Eds.), *Career transitions in turbulent times.* Greensboro, NC: ERIC/CASS Publications.

Miller-Tiedeman, A., & Tiedeman, D. V. (1983). Career? Simply life's gift. In *Proceedings of the 1983 Assembly to Advance Career.* Vista, CA: Lifecareer® Foundation.

Milne, A. A. (1926). *Winnie-the-Pooh.* New York: Dutton.

Prigogine, I. (1980). *From being to becoming: Time and complexity in the physical sciences.* New York: Freeman.

Prigogine, I., & Stengers, I. (1984). *Order out of chaos.* New York: Bantam Books.

Reason, P., & Rowan, J. (Eds). (1981). *Human inquiry: A sourcebook of new paradigm research.* New York: Wiley.

Rulon, P., Tiedeman, D., Tatsuoka, M., & Langmuir, C. R. (1967). *Multivariate statistics for personnel classification.* New York: Wiley.

Swimme, B. (1984). *The universe is a green dragon.* Santa Fe, NM: Bear.

Tiedeman, D. V., & O'Hara, R. P. (1963). *Career development: Choice and adjustment.* New York: College Entrance Examination Board.

Wilber, K. (Ed.). (1982). *Holographic paradigm and other paradoxes.* Boston: Shambhala.

Zohar, D. (1990). *The quantum self: Human nature and consciousness defined by the New Physics.* New York: Morrow.

Zukav, G. (1979). *The dancing wu li masters: An overview of the New Physics.* New York: Morrow.

CHAPTER FIVE

The Lifecareer®¹ Process Theory
A Healthier Choice

Anna Miller-Tiedeman
Lifecareer® Foundation

LIVING LIFE-AS-CAREER nourishes like a good dinner and touches like a gentle wind if we only trust our experience and its learnings. Treating life-as-career provides an easy, convenient, and healthy approach to life direction, which suggests that

- Life, not job, is career.
- Cooperating with the approaching forces while scoping the situation reduces stress and increases motivation.
- Change offers perpetual uncertainty, which provides surprise and newness.
- Less is more.
- Listening to our inner guidance—intelligence, experience, and intuition—will let us know what to do next, even if that's nothing.
- Life is self-organizing.
- Life goes both left and right, and both directions provide equally important information.
- Each person experiences reality created each moment.
- The *now* is seldom problematic.

This chapter introduces the Lifecareer Theory, along with discussion about decision making, wholeness, and the inherent paradigm shift. Career is impotent when treated as something out there in your life to be planned, pursued, and reached. But it is vital when considered in the here and now.

Four propositions suggest how to make living life-as-career easier. This is followed by a discussion of the Lifecareer ethic and suggested possible uses in public education. Most frequently asked questions are then answered. Finally, this chapter holds health as the important outcome.

LITERATURE THAT INSPIRED THE LIFECAREER THEORY

LIFECAREER®: *The Quantum Leap into a Process Theory of Career* (Miller-Tiedeman, 1988) takes off from core concepts of quantum physics, as noted in Capra (1982), Zukav (1979), Wolfe (1981), Bohm (1980), and Prigogine (1980) because "compelling parallels exist between the reality of the microscopic physical world and the social level of our everyday human experience. We're merely larger, more complex composites of the atomically small. From particles to humans, we're all part of the life process functioning in similar process although in different guises" (Miller-Tiedeman, 1989, p. 62). Its new science foundation makes Lifecareer a first attempt to put life in career and give career life, the essential complementarity of the quantum phenomenon.

Complementarity and its accompanying uncertainty principle along with self-organizing systems theory form the process careering foundation, along with Buckminster Fuller's notion that both the right and left of things (what some call *wrong*) helps life advance (Wagschal, 1979). These ideas are used philosophically, not mathematically.

Why wasn't career theory literature used? Primarily because it does not mention process careering or consider the individual as theory maker. Traditional career reflects the worldview it grew up in—Newtonian. Its first and major focus emphasizes adolescent vocational choice—occupational information for the school-to-work transition. Krumboltz and Ranieri (1996) call it the "learn, yearn, and earn" paradigm. Self-sufficiency is sought in a regimen of teaching better, best, and wise decision making about these transitions. This mentality suggests getting your square-peg self into that right-occupational hole, not surfing the process. Research on such things as real-world accuracy (Walls, Fullmer, & Dowler, 1996), vocational maturity, and the like reflects the worldview. So science proved to be the only discipline large enough to handle the Lifecareer idea.

Just as classical physics is a special-case theory in the quantum physics framework, traditional career forms a special case of Lifecareer process theory. You can talk about traditional career with the Lifecareer paradigm, but you cannot do the reverse because traditional career makes very different assumptions. For instance, it defines career as job, supports changing careers, and places the client in a subservient position. This suggests that personal reality lacks the power of conventional wisdom. This perspective fails to recognize that the individual's career theory supersedes those developed by career theorists. These assumptions are untenable in Lifecareer because they do not support renewal and flow in life. However, the assessment aspect, built on Newtonian assumptions, at various times, with selected people, remains appropriate with the caveat that all occupational areas need exploration.

Lifecareer treats each individual as a whole system interacting within larger systems and their environments. Process anchors these transitional systems *ad infinitum*. The Newtonian reductionistic career paradigms such as Super's life roles (in Super, Savickas, & Super, 1996) do not serve as maps of *personal theories* that individuals can use to go from A to B to C in their everyday career developing. For instance, after graduate school, I sent out sixty résumés—and received thirty rejections. Does self-concept theory or life-span discourse matter in my day-to-day life? Absolutely not; I care most about myself within the context of my own career theory. Why? Because I need both to support myself and to have a theory that works for me daily, not a theory or theories professionals use for academic discussion.

In *The Turning Point*, Capra (1982) suggests that the problems biologists cannot solve today—apparently due to their narrow, fragmented approach—all seem to result from treating holistic systems and their interactions with their environment in a reductionist manner. Similarly, career development theorists and professionals today consider first jobs, occupational choice, decision making, and school-to-work transition separately, not holistically. In contrast, the Lifecareer Theory considers the individual to be a living, interactive system that provides self-correcting information. This approach offers the individual an opportunity to become his or her own theory maker. The individual as theory maker, not the theorist handing down his or her version, represents a shift in paradigm.

Each individual life epitomizes a self-organizing system. When relaxing into that system, the individual can make interpretations, and choices follow accordingly. Self-organizing systems theory notes that all living organisms constantly engage in self-renewal with the opportunity to move beyond current boundaries. When individuals identify their self-organizing systems experience, they leap into life's flow effortlessly. With it comes a better functioning immune system, accruing many health benefits. Then living life-as-career becomes as easy as breathing.

THE LIFECAREER BEGINNING

The idea that life is career occurred to me as I watched secondary school students either racing to identify a career or feeling bad because they could not do so during high school. I saw college graduates unable to find work in their major, calling what they found a waystation, not a career. Many of these graduates, in search of that elusive career, returned to graduate school and technical schools for retraining. Many who didn't attend college in the first place thought their chances of finding a career were nil. In some instances, this engendered anger, depression, and hopelessness. These feelings led to stress, which we now know kills off immune system cells (more about the career and its stress connection later).

A doctoral student in one of my summer sessions at Johns Hopkins University described the tension release after learning about the Lifecareer theory: "You don't know how excited I am to know that career is something I'm living, not something I may or may not find."

THE IMPORTANCE OF LIFECAREER

Lifecareer frees you from stress, potentially increasing your motivation and creativity, and offers a better functioning immune system. For instance, when you live life-as-career you know you

- Don't have to search for a career; you have one. You don't look for second and third careers or worry about losing a career or finding another one. Outcome: reduced stress.
- Can trust your inner wisdom that comes from your experience, intelligence, and intuition. You feel joy in your own choices, even though some do not work out but instead provide pathways to newness. Outcome: reduced stress.

- Don't have to know what you're doing all the time. Remember that bees head for the nectar but in the process brush the pollen, which when carried to the next flower brings about cross-fertilization. Life sometimes provides this type of surprise result. Outcome: reduced stress.

- Know that life is a career and you work with it, not against it. Outcome: reduced stress.

- Don't have to fit other people's notions of what you should do. You then free up considerable energy for exploration that reveals many new avenues. Outcome: less fear resulting in reduced stress.

- Know you can find ways to support your needs.

- Understand the importance of money management, distinguishing between need and want, knowing how quickly a sure bet can disappear. Outcome: reduced stress.

- Know that spirituality isn't something you must try to bring into your life. It's something that develops naturally as a result of living the wholeness in life. Spirituality resembles development in that you can only offer to others what you've been able to gain yourself. Outcome: reduced stress.

Stress affects all of us, killing off immune cells. It also plays a role in the diseases that develop over time: heart disease, cancer, and cerebrovascular disorders, which are the diseases most prevalent today. Sapolsky (1994) in his book *Why Zebras Don't Get Ulcers* identifies three kinds of stress: (1) survival, which includes worry about predators, starvation, or bodily harm; (2) chronic stress due to drought, famine, or earthquakes, or having to wander several miles each day for food; and (3) psychological and social stress.

The body will organize to handle the first two types of stress, but the third type is a rather recent invention. Research now suggests that stress-related diseases show up because we use our bodies to handle psychological and social stress whereas they were built to respond to acute physical emergencies, not endless worry about mortgages, relationships, promotions, downsizing, job security, and the like.

A stressor upsets the balance in the body, but the anticipation of an event can do the same damage. For instance, pretend someone asked you to keynote a particular meeting. Most likely, you'll experience that stress numerous times, not just at the keynote. Why? As you practice and envision the audience, your body reacts to the message received. So when you feel that twinge of nervousness, your body reacts by suppressing digestion, depressing growth, and decreasing sex drive, thereby putting reproduction on hold and arresting immune activity. Under sustained stress, we don't recognize pain as quickly, but aspects of memory improve. The stress response does what it's supposed to do. Heart rate, blood pressure, and breathing all increase to deliver nutrients and oxygen faster to take care of the emergency.

If you constantly invoke the stress mechanism, you don't store surplus energy. This results in fatigue and susceptibility to disease. Further, constant stress doesn't allow the body to work on long-term building projects as it's *always* in emergency. In short, stress increases your risk of getting diseases that make you sick and overwhelms your defenses if you're already sick. *However, stress doesn't only freeze the immune system for that particular stressor; it also disassembles it, shrinking tissues and destroying cells.* That's serious in the long run, and when your body breaks down, it's too late to fix what could, in many instances, have been prevented (Sapolsky, 1994).

When you live life-as-career, you use the stress response more often for its original intention—handling acute emergencies—because you invoke cooperation, not confrontational or combative behavior, in an effort to control life. By so doing, you build your body's immunity because that immunity doesn't get killed off as often nor does it need to work with inferior cells. If you insist on control, you may win the external battle but lose the internal war. You also learn that the more you cooperate with life, the better you treat your immune system. This translates into fewer colds, headaches, and other minor ailments, not to mention the big ones.

DECISION MAKING AND LIFECAREER

What about decision making in Lifecareer? All living things decide quite naturally. In *How NOT To Make It . . . And Succeed: Life on Your Own Terms* (Miller-Tiedeman, 1989), I treat decision making as a natural process. I suggest that right and left (wrong) decisions carry equal weight. A main core of traditional career is decision making, focusing on better, best, and right decision making using Newtonian reductionism. Early on, I worked on a decision-making program in the Appalachia Education Laboratory in Charleston, West Virginia, where I met David V. Tiedeman. My first conversation with David concerned decision making. I understand improvement and think that most people work toward that, but I don't understand treating the natural process of decision making as something students need to be taught. Why? Because humans make decisions naturally; cells in the human body, even particles, do the same thing. Zohar (1990) relates the rather well-known double slit experiment, in which you see that photons act quite differently depending on whether, before detection, they get the opportunity to pass through one or two slits in a screen. If only one slit is available, they act like a stream of bullets hitting the screen. If two slits are open, they act like waves, passing through both slits and creating their typical interference pattern on the other side. They somehow know which aspect of their double-sided nature is called for and act accordingly.

David winces when I say that he made a career as a decision-making theorist. However, my comments don't discount David's or anyone else's work in decision making. They merely suggest a different point of view. David was interested in the stages of decision making, I in the process of it: two different perspectives. But our common interest has been accommodation of different perspectives.

My interest in process decision making comes from my commitment to health, both individual and social. I watched high school students in decision-making classes, so concerned about right decisions that they blocked out the learning from the decisions that didn't work out (the left ones). They momentarily forgot the value, interest, and surprise present in new information, both good and bad. Stressing about right decisions weakens the immune system. We ought to be doing everything we can to help individuals build more fully functioning immune systems, which will translate into increased motivation, confidence, and self-esteem.

LIFECAREER AND WHOLENESS

Lifecareer advocates a wholeness in which we know we're part of everything. Therefore it is not restricted to career planning, which many others take to be the new goal of career theory. Instead, Lifecareer is *the dynamic, lived-in-the-moment process defined by each person in individual moments*. It moves forward, collecting all kinds of information both internal and external. Its patterns are like crystals tumbling over each other in a kaleidoscope. It acts like all living things. The more you trust your inner wisdom—experience, intelligence, and intuition—the more you learn to value your own career theory. You then attune yourself to your own cues for the next steps in life.

While in the flow, you seek information, you talk to one or several people. Then you internalize the information, work with new ways to use it, and let time (the process) inform your next step. If you flow with the rhythm of life, you'll avoid major stress, feel good while you wait, and enjoy more satisfaction after you decide. In this way, you support your immune system and experience improved health, probably one of the best reasons for living life-as-career.

When you live your own Lifecareer theory, *you* determine what works and what doesn't. The real test of any career theory is, does it work in *your* life? Physicists know this. Capra (1982) says that physicists hold a common and practical attitude: "When you have a certain theory and you think it's not quite sound, mathematically or otherwise, but it works, then you say, 'Well, there must be something to it.' You then use the model and elaborate on it later" (p. 23). That attitude helped Capra return to the scientific community after his timeout to write *The Tao of Physics* (1975) and *The Turning Point* (1982).

THE PARADIGM SHIFT

Honoring your own career theory represents a paradigm shift in career development. But paradigms don't change easily, particularly at the conforming level of development. For instance, several theorists presented papers at the Professional Development Institute in Chicago. As a presenter, I gave my paper on the Lifecareer Theory.

Afterward, while milling around outside the presenting room, I overheard one of the theorists say, "This Lifecareer Theory is crazy." A second theorist said, "Well, it may have some merit, but I've spent my entire life on occupation/job as career and I don't intend to change now." My conviction of both the joy and the sorrow of a pioneering effort intensified when I heard a third comment: "This theory makes no sense. What does she mean, everyone has a career theory? That couldn't possibly be."

These comments reflect a fear of change. Barker (1990), in his video *The Business of Paradigms: Discovering the Future,* says, "It's so easy to say no to a new idea. After all, new ideas cause change. They disrupt the status quo. They create uncertainty." Following the old path requires less work and, in the case of theorists, keeps egos intact.

If career development theorists resist change to a new paradigm, then who makes the shift? The rest of us. We all change each moment. We can't help it. But sometimes people hold on to old paradigms that make them sick. They often land in our biggest, although not well recognized, career redirection centers—hospitals. Even at this point, some would rather fight than change. Others choose more self-awareness, tired of the old and redundant. Even Winnie-the-Pooh had that experience. Remember, he wandered around the spinney of larch trees wondering whose footprints he saw. He felt perplexed and asked Piglet to help him figure it out. Piglet soon tired and left. Then Pooh, even though he was a bear of little brain, placed his foot in the print and discovered it fit (Milne, 1926). Humans sometimes do this: They go around the conformity bush until they tire, and then it dawns on them what they're doing, so they finally start their journey to a new awareness.

On the other hand, a large number of people make it through life quite well without career counseling or attention to any theory. Many accomplished people continually show us how to listen to our own drummer (career theory) even though they probably don't know that the field of career development exists. Those people may feel greater urgency to rise to their highest potential. For instance, Ilya Prigogine traveled the outskirts of scientific acceptance for twenty years and then in 1977 received the Nobel Prize in chemistry, largely for his dissipative structures theory (Interview, 1983).

People who find it easiest to value their own career theory either seek a greater awareness or they do it naturally anyway. They come from many different socioeconomic levels and possess many different physical abilities. Both these groups cooperate with the approaching forces because they know it will bring new learning. Most likely a significant number of counselors, fed up with trying to orchestrate the current career theories, now work from their own career theory. They Lifecareer naturally, as do many people, and are more likely to work with the client's career theory. As a result, their immune systems function better.

THE LIFECAREER PERSPECTIVE

Life-as-career works differently for each of us. Sometimes a simple incident like attending a concert can change your entire life. Gilbert Kaplan, a former Wall Street journalist and businessman, graduated from Duke University in economics and made his first million by the age of thirty as founder and publisher of *Institutional Investor* magazine. One day, he attended a concert and heard Mahler's Second Symphony. He felt so overcome that immediately afterward he began studying the score of the symphony with a Juilliard instructor and for seven months spent five hours a day conducting a recording by George Solti, memorizing every nuance because he couldn't read music. In 1994, Britain's *Sunday Times* voted Kaplan's upbeat recording of Mahler's Fifth Symphony record of the year. Kaplan still conducts Mahler's works and reports more love for conducting each day ("The Mountain Paradise . . . ," 1984). That one evening at the concert hall changed Kaplan's life even though it appeared a leisure activity. What odds of success would a career counselor have given Kaplan, a man who couldn't even sight-read music?

On the other hand, what feels right sometimes ends in tragedy. Seven-year-old Jessica Dubroff loved flying and wanted to break the existing world record. She followed her bliss, but when her plane took off, it climbed 400 feet, then nosedived into the ground. She lost her life. Her mother said afterward that she would not have made any different decision concerning Jessica's interest in flying. She remarked that after all, Jessica died doing what she loved. And after all, isn't life itself a chance (Sarche, 1996)?

Sometimes you do what you believe and it works over the long run but leaves you ill and broke. That's what happened to Congressman Carl Elliott. Instead of riding the wave of segregation hysteria, he took a moderate position, which in the 1960s proved difficult. Elliott fought for legislation enabling poor students to attend college, for Medicare, and for raising the minimum wage. He says that at that time you couldn't stay in Congress unless you voted against civil rights. But he voted for civil rights and other legislation for the disadvantaged. During his 1964 campaign, right-wing extremists led by the Ku Klux Klan went after Elliott and successfully thwarted his reelection. Two years later, he staked all his money on the governor's race. It left him totally broke. He later said he regretted the debt but not the cause. In 1994, Elliott received the first Kennedy Library Foundation Profile in Courage Award, which came with a $25,000 stipend.

Frequently students major in a field in which they never find work. At other times, they find work in a field for which they have no training or expertise and end up liking it better than the field in which they trained. Life has all kinds of twists and turns. As Lewis Thomas said, "I had no idea I'd end up an essayist and if a medical-journal editor hadn't suggested nine years ago that I try a regular column, I might never have started serious writing. Further, I grew up knowing I wanted to be a doctor, but I didn't know I'd go into research until I nearly finished medical school." Then the war came, and Thomas accepted an assignment to the Rockefeller Institute medical research team (Leishman, 1980, p. 104).

One childhood experience sent Ray Bradbury on what turned into a life of successful writing. It started with Edgar Allan Poe. As Bradbury tells it, he fell in love with Poe's verbal jewelry. From the age of twelve, he began to imitate him and continued until age eighteen. He attributes his success to Poe, William Burroughs, the comics, the carnival and circus people in northern Illinois, and old radio programs. However, he says, Mr. Electrico permanently marked his life. (He later wrote about it in "Something Wicked This Way Comes.") Mr. Electrico, a carnival performer, came through Bradbury's hometown of Waukegan, Illinois, every autumn and sat in his electric chair each night. Someone would pull a switch and Mr. Electrico would reach out and dub everyone in the front row with the electricity that sizzled from his sword. Fire prickled in his mouth and eyes, and his hair stood on end. When he came to Bradbury, he touched him on the brow and chin and said, "Live forever." Enchanted with Mr. Electrico, Bradbury returned to the circus night after night. He and Mr. Electrico shared philosophies. Mr. Electrico said that he and Bradbury had previously met on the battlefield of the Argonne and Bradbury had died in his arms in World War I in France. Bradbury said he didn't know why Mr. Electrico told him that, but it made a deep impression. Bradbury thought Mr. Electrico may have had a dead son, or maybe no son at all, maybe just lonely, and maybe a jokester. But within three months of his last meeting with Mr. Electrico in 1932, Bradbury began writing full-time and never stopped (Plummer, 1980).

A high school student scored 36 out of 36 on the American College Testing (ACT) Program exam but didn't want to attend college. His parents tried to force him, but he resisted. Finally they relented and he went to work. But two years later, he applied for college admission, got accepted, and four years later graduated. To everything there is a purpose and season (Ecclesiastes 3:1).

Recently Cheyenne Rouse, an artist, embarked on a vacation that changed her life forever. She left balmy Miami and started a tour of the scenic Southwest, which included stops in New Mexico and Utah. The beauty brought tears to her eyes. A few months later, Cheyenne returned to Miami, sold her half of the family clothing store, packed all her earthly goods, and headed to San Diego to start a freelance outdoor photography business. She worked at three jobs until her business took off. Now she makes enough to work only on photography. Her interest in photography started when her father gave her a camera for her fifteenth birthday. She's also discovered that she's in a good field, as many of the outdoor magazine editors complain they don't get enough input from women (O'Hara, 1996).

Each of these stories illustrates life-as-career at work in various circumstances unique to the individual. Each life-as-career looks different. None of these lives can be duplicated. That's why no one else's notion about how to do something or even whether to do something at all usually works. This dovetails with Lewin's life-space idea, in which he suggests that each individual behaves in response to his or her worldview (Lewin, 1951).

Living life-as-career is a cooperative venture with life (all forms). We need to support each other's life journey, not judge it. Support increases confidence, self-esteem, and potentially motivation. It also tends to strengthen the immune system, making us less susceptible to various ailments and diseases.

Cindy Crawford attended DeKalb High School and graduated four years after I left my counseling job there to move to California. Valedictorian of her class, she went on to Northwestern University in Chicago. After one semester, she left to pursue a modeling career in New York. The rest is history, as she's now one of the most famous supermodels in America. Cindy jettisoned an opportunity for a college degree and followed her inner wisdom. But she had support from her hairdresser, makeup artist, personal trainer, image stylist, photographer, designer, caterer, magazine editor, photo editor, and more. Everyone needs support while pursuing his or her dream even when it may not produce such astounding results.

THE LIFECAREER ETHIC[2]

Over the last thirteen years, many people have asked questions about the Lifecareer ethic. In short, its ethic is unbroken wholeness, unfoldment, not revolutionary change. Lifecareer suggests no rupture in reality, but rather steadily changing continuity. In a religious system, there are injunctions—things that should be done and things that should not be done, relating to what is good or evil or undesirable—to improve and prevent whatever the religious system encourages and forbids. In the Lifecareer ethic, anything that encourages the steady and continuous connection between the affective and cognitive, the physical and spiritual, is fostered. Lifecareering supports harmonious development in these four areas. The stories in the preceding section reflect that harmonious flow.

Taking action when anything in life threatens to disrupt this continuous flow exemplifies the ethical imperative. This is not stoicism, total submission to natural law; rather it is active participation in your development. To do this, you reflect with sensitivity—getting new organizations of personal experience and coming up with concept-advancing holistic impressions.

Further, Lifecareer does not have violence in it. It is human development at peace with self. Lifecareer does not have to be earned; it is a gift to everything on Earth. Life is. In Lifecareer unfolding, you exercise responsible stewardship. You don't *own* life. You only *use* it. In Lifecareer, you can control knowledge about and sensitivity to life, but life does not belong to anyone in particular. Responsible stewardship by each individual involves letting life unfold in everyone. Living the Lifecareer ethic requires *strenuous reflection* on where life is going and on all incoming information. You ask, What are the antecedents and direction of life? Based on personal answers to this question, you cooperate and flow with life rather than trying to control it. This can be done without impeding others' career development. Lifecareer is not career development in the selfish sense; it is career development in the higher sense of self—a self spirit in unity with the universe in its entirety, a self continually seeking to know unity wholly. Prigogine (1980) and more recently Zohar (1990) call this *the arrow of time,* which continually works in the chaos of self-organizing systems, dedifferentiating in harmony with continued reintegration in rhythm. When I walk on the beach, I see that rhythm in action. As I walk, I see a large group of seagulls in my walking path. As I approach, they back off. I pass them, and they return to the edge of the water. Perfect orchestration.

In short, Lifecareer is following life nonintrusively. You don't rupture the stream of life. You *are* the stream. You are the current. Your intention is to flow smoothly, divining direction, continually active and alert to all movement.

However, during redefinition and while flowing, the stream is frequently interrupted. In *Women Who Run with the Wolves,* Estes (1992) suggests that wolves that have lost the scent scramble to find it again and look funny in the process. They hop in the air, run in circles, plow up the ground with their noses, scratch the ground, run ahead, then back, and then stand still. It appears they have lost their wits, but actually they are trying to pick up all the clues they can find by biting them down from the air, filling their lungs with scents at ground and shoulder level, and tasting to see who has passed through recently. Their ears rotate like satellite dishes, as if picking up transmissions from afar. Once they have all the clues in place, they know what to do.

Sometimes the redirection process for humans looks as strange as it does for wolves. But they too need to receive all necessary clues in order to know what to do. Sometimes these clues come quickly, but often they are time extended, causing us to believe nothing is working or will work. But in time, situations resolve themselves.

PROPOSITIONS THAT SUPPORT LIVING LIFE-AS-CAREER

The following propositions buttress the life-direction process:

Proposition 1. Life is self-organizing. Self-organizing systems theory, an integral part of today's quantum physics, acknowledges that order comes from chaos—specifically, that the more coherent a system becomes, the more susceptible it is to falling apart. The breakout of freedom in Eastern Europe and the dissipation of the U.S.S.R. serve as prime examples, as does our current downsizing problem.

Believing that life is self-organizing means putting energy into cooperating with life, not controlling it. Ilya Prigogine, the Nobel-winning chemist, pioneered the "dissipative structures" concept. He describes them as open systems that maintain their structure by continually exchanging energy with their environment (Lukas, 1980). According to Prigogine, fluctuation is the main process element of all self-organization. Self-organizing living systems experience countless fluctuations. Periodically, fluctuations are driven to their limits. This imbalance is frequently called *stress*. During such imbalance, two possibilities exist: maintenance/renewal (a restoring) or growth (a transition). Because all living things experience fluctuations, they constantly strive for balance by maintaining and/or growing. For instance, walking fast or running causes the heart to beat more rapidly and breathing to be faster and deeper. When the activity is stopped, heart and breath return to normal. The body resumes its normal rhythm; it is maintaining. However, Prigogine (Interview, 1983) suggests that living organisms are always far from equilibrium.

On the other hand, during crisis periods, when nothing seems to work—for instance, when you're caught in downsizing, divorce, or business failure—you try to maintain balance, to regain the former equilibrium. But the fluctuations may be too great, and instability results. Then you experience mental and/or physical uncertainty, which can show up in the body, the behavior, and/or social and professional relationships. Physical and mental symptoms such as depression, headaches, or other problems can arise, reflecting a depressed immune system. You may feel as if your life is standing still, which often results in low physical energy, requiring more sleep and perhaps less socializing. But after a while, the system reorganizes and either maintains at a new level or reaches a breakthrough. One woman reported that she knows she's close to a breakthrough when she feels most confused and blocked. If she can live through that confusion, she experientially knows that something new will emerge.

In attaining this new state, a self-organizing system has grown and learned. It is different now and has the opportunity to experience more stability. This also happens after a serious illness, when people report they're not the same as they were before. They have grown, they have evolved, they feel healthier than they did before the illness. Sometimes the system cannot adapt to such challenges. If it does not adapt or does not do so quickly enough, then it will continue on as before or wither.

A story in Ann Landers' column illustrates how life continues to self-organize. Two sisters wrote Ann about their eighty-three-year-old mother. After her second husband died, she decided to move into a retirement home. The sisters usually visited their mom on Sundays, but they decided to visit her on her birthday, which fell on a Wednesday. They baked her a birthday cake and drove over to the retirement home. They decided to go straight to her room. When they opened the door, they found their mom in her negligee on the sofa necking up a storm with an eighty-four-year-old resident whose wife had died the previous year. Mom, surprised, quickly blurted out, "It's OK. Eddy and I plan to get married" (Landers, 1996).

Mom didn't have to plan getting involved; all she had to do was cooperate with the approaching forces while checking out the situation. She could have refused the advances, but that didn't feel right. Further, mom in her wisdom probably understood the Ecclesiastes verse that to everything there is a time, season, and purpose.

Life abhors disorganization, children's rooms in chaos notwithstanding. Life continually self-organizes dependably, even at the particle level. Bodily cells, organs, groups, communities, states, nations, world, universe, and even individual Lifecareers—all self-organize. They can't help it. It's built into the system, as life's career is renewal. Now this doesn't necessarily mean that we always like the results. It merely means that self-organization is built into life—and is continuous. So when you fail to organize, life does it for you. And even when you do organize, life often puts its own spin on that organization. How many times have you thought you would do something, and a phone call, a knock on the door, or a toilet spillover changed your plans? Life happens without our permission.

When you trust life and know that it works, not always the way you want it to, but it works, then you relax and let your career develop naturally because you know that life will continue to inform you about necessary changes. This is markedly different from traditional career theories that suggest you can control life, along with the needed prescription to make it, and accompanying plans and goals. These theories come with a preponderance for living in the future. In contrast, Lifecareerists cooperate with life, with the approaching forces, making appropriate decisions in the moment. When you live life-as-career, you may not need a career plan, as following inner wisdom—experience, intelligence, and intuition—and organizing, not career planning and goal setting, are the dominant activities. You therefore need to stay in touch with your experience, intelligence, and intuition. In order to cooperate with the approaching forces, you seek appropriate information when necessary. The orientation is flexibility and flow while continually living in the *now*. This does not suggest letting life happen without thought. It affirms the close attention to your inner wisdom and taking action when necessary—the basic process of being intelligent.

Motion constitutes the basic self-organizing systems activity, and motion is the central dynamic in Lifecareer. "For every (re)action occurring in nature, some change in either mass or energy occurs" (Milani & Smith, 1985, p. 148). Even when the overall system remains stable and seems to produce no perceivable change, change happens.

Internal and external forces co-create change and produce changes that must, by definition, affect all. This is difficult for many to accept as they often view certain changes within themselves as being forced on them because others refuse to change. For instance, I'd like to change my life, but I'm locked in by society's rules. If I had my choice, I'd . . . This implies that an individual is being forced to do something against his or her will. "Inasmuch as an individual refuses to accept the choice to change, he or she limits society's ability to change" (Milani & Smith, 1985, p. 148). Because everything is connected, waiting for others to set you free or to make a way for you is counterproductive. "Rotationally, the only way to change any part of society is to change the self first" (p. 148). However, any one change shuffles the entire universe in some way, as it is a web of relationships.

Proposition 2. Guiding from inner wisdom using intentions. In using your inner wisdom, it's helpful to ask yourself if the information is culturally mandated—what the majority agree is true—or placed there by you, as that information dictates your choices. As you think about that, consider that from birth your parents tell you how it is; then on to school, where teachers not only tell you how they think it is but also suggest you learn how others think it is; and then on to church, where the rabbi/minister/priest dictates his or her reality version. Not knowing two realities exist—personal and common—and not getting much practice in discerning the two, you're denied the option to consciously choose either, as you have to be aware that a choice exists in order to deliberately make it. So you might want to question the information that comes to you, asking, does it still work? Or does it need updating?

In considering what you believe about inner wisdom, remember that experience, intelligence, and intuition combined form a more powerful information source than what is collectively agreed upon by others. You might call that your cosmic Internet. If you don't log on, you miss out on the information.

In order to log on, you need quiet time. Meditation offers a good way to tune into your cosmic Internet. It's relaxing and healthy. Benson (1975) at Harvard University discovered this when he studied transcendental meditators. He found meditation, or the relaxation response, can lower blood pressure and reduce drug use. Benson suggests that many different meditation approaches can elicit the relaxation response, producing health benefits. Tests at the Thorndike Memorial Laboratory at Harvard showed that similar technique used with any sound, phrase, prayer, or mantra brings forth the same physiologic changes noted during transcendental meditation: decreased oxygen consumption; decreased carbon-dioxide elimination; decreased rate of breathing. In other words, any one of the age-old or newly devised techniques produces the same physiologic results. Benson said, "We claim no innovation but simply scientific validation of age-old wisdom" (p. 114). So even if you're not interested in listening to your inner wisdom, you might want to try meditation or the relaxation response for health reasons.

When you surf life's process, consider using goals for such things as joy and peace. That way, you don't have a time constraint, which often creates anxiety when the goal isn't met. Further, you don't lose energy trying to determine why it didn't work. That rehearsal time could be used on something else. Chopra (1987) suggests that what you attend to grows and produces new energy. This attention on goals places your awareness in a narrow channel, and the river of life runs more broadly. Furthermore, the highest state of attention goes beyond goals and anchors internally with a balance between rest and activity. Both goal-setting and traditional career attitudes encourage activity, with little focus on rest. Without the rests in music, little melody would emerge. The same thing holds true for career developing.

So what is the alternative? Try setting intentions without time designations. Play with your intentions. Forget them. Remember them. Place them in a different order of priority. But return to them until you're sure they hold no meaning for you. Some people carry hundreds of intentions on their computer calendar. What seems a hot intention over time turns cold and vice versa. But by listing the intention, you don't lose it. Further, you'll discover that when your intentions are one with life's rhythm, the answers manifest quickly. When they're not, the answers take longer and in some instances don't come at all. If you want to, track your intentions: Write "Intention" on the left side of the paper and "Date Completed" on the right side. Often when you set an intention, you don't have any idea how to go about it. But if you keep it in your attention, ideas will start popping into your mind. Write them down on paper and place them in a folder, or log them on your computer.

It also works in reverse. Sometimes ideas come to you from time to time. If you keep them filed, you may discover that a book emerges. The Lifecareer Theory came that way. I didn't set out to write a theory. I started with ideas on paper slips. I then said, "I think this would make a book." *How NOT To Make It . . . And Succeed* was born. *LIFECAREER®: The Quantum Leap into a Process Theory of Career* also first appeared on paper slips, as did my subsequent books.

This leads to a comment about style. You may be the type who sits down and writes a book. Or you may outline first. It all depends on your style. That's another reason to pay attention to your life-as-career developing: to observe your workstyle.

Proposition 3. Lifecareer honors both right and left decisions. Acknowledging both the right and left in life precludes agonizing over wise or right decision making. Buckminster Fuller (Wagschal, 1979) notes that people don't talk about walking on their right and wrong foot; they talk about the right and left foot; and that works quite well and efficiently. No "right" decisions exist, only decisions that you like better than others. All decisions count in life. Those that go left teach us the most.

For instance, Karl Pribram, the famous neurosurgeon, has been criticized by more conventional neuroscientists for his bold speculations and for seizing upon new findings outside his field in an effort to understand memory. Pribram recalls the pioneer memory researcher Ewald Hering's remark that suggests every scientist at some point in his or her work has to risk "looking foolish."

The scientist begins to be interested in his or her work and what the findings mean. Then, says Pribram, as quoted in Wilber,

[H]e has to choose. If he starts to ask questions and tries to find answers to understand what it all means, he will look foolish to his colleagues. On the other hand, he can give up the attempt to understand what it all means; he won't look foolish and he'll learn more and more about less and less. (Wilber, 1982, p. 19)

Pribram concludes that you need the courage to look foolish. In Lifecareer, reading and following your inner wisdom could somewhere along the way require the courage to look foolish as well as the courage to continue regardless of what others say.

The part of life that doesn't work creates occupations both for us to work in and to be served by. Imagine how many people would be unemployed if tomorrow morning the world turned perfect.

Proposition 4. We monitor the reality that creates itself for us. Therefore, each person lives his or her own mythology. Realizing that reality creates itself each moment in our heads precludes allowing others to define that reality. Others include parents, teachers, counselors, friends, career theorists, and the like. This belief also precludes trying to create reality for someone else. Someone else includes those just mentioned and especially clients.

The shift in how we consider reality comes from quantum physics. The universe is made up of waves and particles. A major switch in physics occurred when physicists realized that individual scientists looking for a particle found a particle; when others looked for a wave, they found a wave. In other words, objectivity fell from grace in the scientific field. Zukav (1979) quotes John Wheeler, the well-known physicist at Princeton, who notes that *participator* replaces the term *observer* of classical theory, the person who stands safely behind the thick glass wall and watches without taking part. "It can't be done, quantum mechanics says" (p. 54).

However, professors still ask students to be objective as if objectivity is possible. But it is not. No one knows what anyone else ought to do, nor does anyone know how the transformation we now experience will affect our lives.

On the other hand, as Zohar (1990) suggests, we can objectively agree that a cat won't turn into a kangaroo. But five of us can watch an accident and tell different stories about what happened. So we need to approach the idea of objectivity with caution.

To practice taking responsibility for your perceptions, ask yourself how you feel about this chapter. If you like it, that's you. If you don't, that too is you. The chapter provides a mirror for you to reexamine your value system and career theory. This applies to anything you experience. For instance, I've heard people say (as I too said before I caught on to being a part of what I observe), "What a boring speaker." I now realize the speaker is neither inherently boring nor interesting. It all depends on what fits with my values, beliefs, and personal criteria.

At the 1995 ACA Convention in Denver, I was amazed at the opening speaker's finger pointing, shouting, and unilateral viewpoint on multiculturalism. But I commented, "That approach doesn't work for me." Further, I came home and wrote a paper about it, using development as a framework. When you recognize you can't separate yourself from what you observe, your language changes from verbal attacks to owning your own position. At this point, you recognize that what you don't like goes counter to your values and beliefs and what you do like agrees with them.

Proposition 5. Stay in the now. If you do, you'll never have a moment you can't handle. Forecasting frequently causes problems. This works in all aspects of life. For instance, in May 1990, when I had to decide whether to take David to the emergency room, my inner wisdom, not the doctor, informed me, and the *now* worked. When I sat through two major operations within four days, each moment worked. Living through the intensive care situation with ninety days of stable and holding, I found the *now* worked. At the end of this episode, I looked back and wondered how I survived. Then I remembered that I stayed in the *now*. That's true for any aspect of life, even death. It's only the *thought* of death that frightens us. We'll all probably do just fine when our moment arrives.

PRINCIPLES FOR WORKING WITH LIFECAREER IN PUBLIC EDUCATION AND CAREER COUNSELING

There are three major principles to follow in applying these concepts to career counseling.

Principle 1. Abandon judgment. Otherwise, you'll make statements such as, "This student is disorganized and has poor decision strategies." One person's disorganization is another's organization, and who's to say that someone else's strategies aren't good? This question clearly shows the assumptions the counselor quickly makes and the role he or she takes, which is evaluative. Perhaps in the professional's value system, the student doesn't quite measure up, but that doesn't say anything about the student.

Ilya Prigogine says, "Nature is part of us and we are part of it. We can recognize ourselves by the description we give to it" (Lukas, 1980, p. 88). This means the counselor finds the student's organization and decision-making strategy values different from her or his own. In Lifecareer counseling (quantum counseling), you recognize you cannot separate yourself from what you're observing, even when you're observing students.

Principle 2. Consider decision making a natural phenomenon. Although I think students gain from any educational class, I prefer to see decision making taught using process examples. You could start, for instance, by using the body and nature as examples. Six trillion reactions occur each second in our bodies (Chopra, 1987). That represents rather rapid decision making, and without formal instruction. I would like students to know that each cell in the body knows what to do. For instance, if you transplant heart cells into another organ, they migrate back to the heart, suggesting that heart cells don't long to be lung cells. It's not about knowing your place; it's about understanding your destiny. Those living organisms without the ability to reason do much better than we humans!

Desert Solitaire (Abbey, 1968) tells about the yucca tree, which is fertilized by a moth, not by bees or hummingbirds:

> The moth lays its eggs in the ovary of the yucca flower where the larvae, as they develop, feed on the growing seeds, eating enough to reach maturity, but leaving enough in the pod to allow the plant, with the help of the desert winds, to sow next year's yucca crop. In return for this nursery care, the moth transfers the yucca's flower pollen from anther to pistil, thus accomplishing pollination. (pp. 25–26)

There are many other wonderful examples of the naturalness of decision making when you start seeing it from a process perspective.

Principle 3. Encourage living from the inside out, not the reverse. When you do this, you'll encourage development. Additionally, it relaxes you and removes the necessity of responding to something that's perhaps not meant for you. Williamson (1994) summarizes it best: "We're not so much trying to make a place for ourselves in the world; we're trying to make a place in ourselves for the world" (p. 40).

Living from your inner wisdom involves trial and error. People can offer advice and suggestions, but the greatest learning comes with trial and error. Rejoice in this, as it's the way life works. Anytime you parallel the life process, you end up winning. Reno Dulbecco (1987), a Nobel prize winner in medicine, says that it may seem that life aims at specific goals. But detailed analysis suggests no grand plan; the result occurs through trial and error. "The only beauty of this approach is that it works. This is a fundamental aspect of life; associations are established however possible through the use of a great hodgepodge of clues, signals, molecules. *Associations that work are retained, others are thrown away. Life is pragmatic; it recognizes only success*" (p. 451, emphasis added).

So start by supporting all kinds of exploration, even those you think won't work for the student. Let go of trying to save students from their experience. This increases student confidence. Set your main goal to help students find value and feel comfortable with all of their decisions. Further, let's not make a judgment even in the recesses of our mind about poor strategies or disorganization or anything else, because this information gets communicated. Our thoughts travel on the electromagnetic band and communicate nonverbally to our clients. This nonverbal information may pose a barrier depending on the client's awareness. It also dams up creativity and tends to hinder life directions. I don't think we professionals realize the damaging effect of our negative thoughts nor the incredible enabling effect of our positive ones.

Let's pretend a student scored 36 out of 36 on the ACT and wants to drive a truck and delay college. What would you do? Well, you'd better support the student's notions, because none of us, including parents, have a lock on anyone's future. Further, we ought to admit that to our clients. Whatever the student's choice, you want to make certain to support the student's career theory and individual notions. That way, you keep all options open for the student. In addition, you don't want to introduce doubt that could cost the student hours, days, weeks, or months of nonaction or even result in giving up a dream. In essence, you want to give your student's career theory the right environment in which to develop and grow.

These three principles in turn suggest eight specific ways to provide helpful counseling:

1. *Tell your students up front that they have a career: It's life.* Clearing this up at the beginning helps the student at least start out not feeling behind. Listen to how the student discusses future earning activity. In the mid-80s, I started hearing more and more students talk about

starting their own business. That thought should be encouraged. Follow the flow of student thought, interrupting here and there with bits of information that may prove helpful. For instance, anyone who lives in the United States ought to know that jobs will come and go, be downsized in and out, and be outsourced when possible. Second, most of the ladders in the corporate world have been damaged or eliminated—another reason why you want to anchor people in their inner wisdom.

A gentle, uninterrupted flow imprints a good, secure feeling in the body. As a result, endorphins are released, creating possibility for more motivation and confidence, thereby increasing self-esteem.

2. *Assure your students that they know best how or if something is working.*

3. *Encourage trial and error without judgment.* How else do we discover our potential?

4. *Make sure that even though a student measures highest in, say, business, that he or she looks at the other occupational areas as well.* We choose what we know. In addition, more technical occupations might become options with improved basic math skills. So encourage multiple exploration. Ultimately the student will explore what feels right in the moment, or maybe not explore at all, which is OK. Many people learn through experience, so maybe your student will have to explore many areas through job experience. Some counselors and parents jump to the conclusion that learning through experience is a waste of time. However, it's only a waste to onlookers; it serves the individual in the experience quite well. So we have to first convince ourselves we can let go of our notions of "expert" and invite the individual to assume that role. This means abandoning the age-old notion of objectivity and supporting subjective data.

5. *Allow for decision-making experience over time by encouraging three- and four-year plans.* Students can modify these plans each semester as their experience changes. That way they see their decision making applied to important situations.

6. *Make sure the student understands that his or her internal information is primary, more important than what shows up on the test.* Lifecareer holds that humans are intelligent and would get along even if career development didn't exist. This doesn't mean counselors can't be helpful.

They can. But they must change the basis on which they help. They need to support their clients' individual journeys, helping them over major barriers. This, in my opinion, would provide work for counselors for a long time to come.

7. *Let students observe your enthusiasm for change.* Educate them about how all situations have opportunity in them. Feel excitement, not fear, about the future. However you feel about change will be communicated to the student.

8. *Encourage students to focus on action, not outcome.* This will make for a happier camper, a healthier immune system, and greater potential for moving ahead.

CONCLUSION

Living life-as-career is an effortless and cooperative venture. Our need to control and our inattention to life's desire gets in our way. Reynolds (1984), in his book *Playing Ball on Running Water,* suggests that our solutions to our problems come when we merge with them, adapt, and accept them for what they are. He tells how Constantin Stanislavsky, former director of the Moscow Art Theater and pioneer of Method acting, suggests to actors that their goal in acting, whether on stage or in life, isn't perfect control of their surroundings or their feelings, nor inspiration, nor transcendent experience. "The goal is simply learning to do what one can, leaving nature to bring about some results from the action. One gives up one's self in the doing and accepts the consequences as data for determining the next doing" (p. 91). That's the optimal attitude for living life-as-career.

In the final analysis, we'll all move toward Lifecareering, return to our bodies, and start learning what it's like to be more fully human. Then we'll ask ourselves, Why did it take so long? And we'll remember, *It's the journey.*

After a time of decay comes the turning point. The powerful light, once banished, returns. Movement comes about naturally, arising spontaneously. For this reason the transformation of the old becomes easy. The old is discarded and the new introduced. Both measures accord with the time; therefore no harm results.
—*adapted from the* I Ching

NOTES

1. Lifecareer and Life-Is-Career are registered trademarks of the Lifecareer Foundation.

2. In 1984, while teaching a summer class in Lifecareer at Loyola College, Professor Lee Richmond, my sponsor, arranged for me to lunch with Dr. Beatrice Sarlos, professor of philosophy at Loyola College. She had read *How NOT To Make It . . . And Succeed,* and I invited her comments. They proved a rare gift and burned themselves into my memory. So I gratefully credit Professor Sarlos for her teachings. However, the section represents my memory of that conversation, for which I take full responsibility.

REFERENCES

Abbey, E. (1968). *Desert solitaire.* New York: Touchstone.

Bach, R. (1977). *Illusions: The adventures of a reluctant messiah.* New York: Dell/Eleanor Friede.

Barker, J. (1990). *The Business of paradigms: Discovering the future* [Video]. Burnsvine, MN: Charthouse International Learning Corporation.

Benson, H. (1975). *The relaxation response.* New York: Morrow.

Bohm, D. (1980). *Wholeness and the implicate order.* London: Routledge.

Capra, F. (1975). *The tao of physics.* Boston: Shambhala.

Capra, F. (1982). *The turning point: Science, society, and the rising culture.* New York: Simon & Schuster.

Capra, F. (1983). The turning point. In C. Lynch, A. Miller-Tiedeman, and D. V. Tiedeman (Eds.), *Proceedings of the 1983 Assembly to Advance Career,* Vista, CA: Lifecareer® Foundation.

Chopra, D. (1987). *Creating health: How to wake up the body's intelligence.* Boston: Houghton Mifflin.

Dulbecco, R. (1987). *The design of life.* Quebec, Canada: McGill University Press.

Estes, C. P. (1992). *Women who run with the wolves.* New York: Ballantine.

Ferguson, M. (1980). *The aquarian conspiracy.* Los Angeles: Tarcher.

Fuller, B. (1981). Critical path. New York: St. Martin's.

Interview. Ilya Prigogine. *Omni,* May 1993.

Krumboltz, J. and Ranieri, A. (1996). Learn, yearn, and earn. In R. Feller and G. Walz (Eds.), *Career transitions in turbulent times.* Greensboro, NC: ERIC/CASS Publications.

Landers, A. (1996, April 14). Elderly mom finds fiancé, stuns kids. *North County Times.*

Leishman, K. (1980, May). Interview with Lewis Thomas: Like other animals, we go around creating whatever reality we perceive. *Quest.*

Lewin, K. (1951). *Field theory in social science.* New York: HarperCollins.

Lukas, M. (1980). The world according to Ilya Prigogine. *Quest.*

Milani, M., & Smith, B. R. (1985). *Rotational physics: The principles of energy.* Westmoreland, NH: Fanshaw.

Miller-Tiedeman, A. (1988). *LIFECAREER®: The quantum leap into a process theory of career.* Vista, CA: Lifecareer® Foundation.

Miller-Tiedeman, A. (1989). *How not to make it . . . and succeed: The truth about your lifecareer.* Vista, CA: Lifecareer® Foundation.

Miller-Tiedeman, A. (1992). *LIFECAREER®: How it can benefit you*. Vista, CA: Lifecareer® Foundation.

Milne, A. A. (1926). *Winnie-the-Pooh*. New York: Dutton.

The mountain paradise that was Mahler's hell. (1994, July 29–August 4). *The European*.

O'Hara, T. (1996, April 22). Del Mar artist captures West on film. *North County Times*.

Plummer, W. (1980, June). Interview with Ray Bradbury: The biggest influence on my life in that magical year was Mr. Electrico. *Quest*.

Prigogine, I. (1980). *From being to becoming: Time and complexity in the physical sciences*. New York: Freeman.

Reynolds, D. (1984) *Playing ball on running water*. New York: Quill.

Sapolsky, R. (1994). *Why zebras don't get ulcers: A guide to stress, stress-related diseases, and coping*. New York: Freeman.

Sarche, J. (1996, April 12). Young pilot dies in stormy crash. *North County Times*.

Super, D., Savickas, M. L., & Super, C. M. (1996). The life-span, life-space approach to careers. In D. Brown and L. Brooks (Eds.), *Career choice and development*. (3rd ed.). San Francisco: Jossey-Bass.

Swimme, B. (1984). *The universe is a green dragon*. Santa Fe, NM: Bear.

Wagschal, P. H. (1979). *The education of Buckminster Fuller*. Amherst: University of Massachusetts Press.

Walls, R. T., Fullmer, S. L., & Dowler, S. L. (1996, March). Functional vocational cognition: Dimensions of real-world accuracy. *The Career Development Quarterly, 44*.

Wilber, K. (Ed.). (1982). *Holographic paradigm and other paradoxes*. Boston: Shambhala.

Williamson, M. (1994). *Illuminata: Thoughts, prayers, rites of passage*. New York: Random House.

Wolfe, F. A. (1981). *Taking the quantum leap: The new physics for non-scientists*. New York: HarperCollins.

Zohar, D. (1990). *The quantum self*. New York: Morrow.

Zukav, G. (1979). *The dancing wu li masters*. New York: Morrow.

CHAPTER SIX

How Does "God-Talk" Speak to the Workplace?

An Essay on the Theology of Work

Harvey L. Huntley, Jr.
Lutherans in Mission Parish

Work is a topic capable of generating considerable discussion. One reason, no doubt, is that for a majority of adults, work occupies a substantial proportion of their waking hours. Particularly in modern America, a person's work is a dominant factor in identity—both for the individual and for the wider society (Bellah, Madsen, Sullivan, Swidler, & Tipton, 1985). Any human activity that commands so much time, energy, and interest is a fertile arena for theological reflection.

From a theological standpoint, a key issue in work is its meaning. For many people in postindustrial society, the meaning of work is a major issue as well. Here are some illustrative cases based on situations with which I have had contact:

B. is an attractive, talented woman in her early forties who has been feeling useless and unfulfilled for several years. Unhappily married to an alcoholic (her second marriage), she began looking for a job about a year ago in hopes that work might give her life a needed focus and purpose. After about nine months in a job that initially appeared promising, she concluded that it is not satisfying and meaningful. Recently she decided to resign her present job and seek a divorce.

D. is a well-educated man in his mid-thirties with a $50,000-a-year job with the United States Postal Service. Although his job is repetitive and uninteresting, he likes the lifestyle it supports and the security it provides. Each week, he literally lives for the weekend when he can retreat to a mountain home with his family. He mainly looks forward to retirement, when he anticipates enjoying a generous pension. A major constraint in his life scenario, however, is that automation is rapidly eliminating many of the jobs that he supervises. It is a real question whether his job will be secure enough, at least in its present form, to carry him until he is eligible for retirement.

Both C. and A. are high school seniors who recently attended a church retreat on career planning. During the retreat, they heard their pastor talk about how work can provide meaning and purpose in life. They both responded with incredulity: "Pastor, nobody believes that stuff anymore. People don't find meaning in their work. Whom are you trying to kid? People just work to get things they want and need in life." Neither C. nor A. has made any decision about a lifework.

E. is a public school teacher in her mid-fifties and a very committed member of her church. Recently the state offered teachers with more than twenty-five years' experience an attractive early retirement option. She pondered the offer for several months before finally deciding to accept it. One of her reasons for the decision is that now she can do things she always wanted to do but never attempted because of work commitments. For the moment, she has no idea as to what she will devote the next ten or more years of her life.

All four of the preceding examples reflect one or more realities prevalent in workplaces of late twentieth-century America. In one form or another, all four pose the issue of the meaning of work. These are not isolated cases. Numerous observers of the contemporary workplace—from sociologists to theologians—have described work as largely void of meaning for most people. At best, work is ambiguous; yet there is a strong desire among workers for meaning in work. Those who do express satisfaction in work claim to find meaning beyond compensation. At the same time, there is considerable discontent in the American workplace, especially among the young. Because of the isolation of workers from the final product of their labor, the confusion between means and ends in work, and the loss of personal feeling in the rational technological workplace, more and more people are questioning the traditional American work ethic and even the necessity of work. Generally, utilitarian ends have justified work; but the meaning of such utility is rarely, if ever, addressed (Arendt, 1958; Nelson, 1954; Terbel, 1972; Bellah, Madsen, Sullivan, Swidler, & Tipton, 1985).

Given such a context for thinking about work, how does Christian theology illumine the meaning of work? How might the insights of theology speak to people like the ones whose situations we have noted? Unfortunately there is no simple and clear-cut answer to such questions. Much of what theologians have said about work is buried in obscure and erudite tomes unlikely to be read or comprehended by many working people. Among contemporary theologians, moreover, there is a fairly broad continuum of views about work. All can be substantiated on biblical grounds in the minds of their proponents. In fact, some theologians use identical biblical texts to bolster radically different views. This chapter summarizes four interpretations of work in contemporary theology:

1. Work as necessity
2. Work as good in itself—a blessing
3. Work as vocation
4. Work as co-creation

The foregoing provide a basis for assessing the theological significance of work and insights that theology offers contemporary workplaces. Following a review of these positions, this chapter identifies some common themes about work and proposes some applications of theological insights for work in contemporary society.

The perspective from which I am writing is obviously limited in terms of spiritual traditions. My intent is not to imply Christian exclusivism or superiority. I am simply recognizing the tradition of my experience and conviction as the spiritual context out of which I speak. It would be presumptuous for me to address the topic of this article from a broader religious perspective, because I am not deeply immersed in other spiritual traditions. Hopefully the reflective method employed here can be adapted by others who represent different spiritual traditions. My base is a Christian one; therefore I have written from that perspective. No doubt, persons interested in work and its meaning could address the theological issues found herein from Jewish, Islamic, Hindu, Buddhist, or other spiritual perspectives. I would deem such offerings an enrichment to the present work, but I do not consider myself qualified by background or experience to attempt such a task.

THE NECESSITY FOR WORK

Widespread among various biblical writers is the view that work is an unavoidable and necessary part of the natural order of creation. Although everyone is expected to work, there is no implication that work is by nature dehumanizing. It is simply a necessary part of the God-given framework of human experience. To be denied work is to be denied one's full humanity (Richardson, 1952). One biblical example is St. Paul's exhortation to the Christians at Thessalonica:

> For even when we were with you, we gave you this command. Anyone unwilling to work should not eat. For we hear that some of you are living in idleness, mere busybodies, not doing any work. Now such persons we command and exhort in the Lord Jesus Christ to do their work quietly and to earn their own living. (2 Thessalonians 3:10–12, New Revised Standard Version)

Among major twentieth-century theologians, Karl Barth (1961) is a strong advocate of the necessity for work. For Barth, work is part of our human obedience to the divine command, but it is not the essence of what God expects or requires of people. Although recognizing the necessity for work, the Bible does not hold it in very high regard. Neither Paul nor Jesus placed much emphasis upon their worldly occupations of tent making and carpentry. Thus for Barth there is virtually no biblical support for the exalted views of work that have characterized much Protestant theology since the Reformation. Barth distinguishes between the work of God as creator and the work of people as creatures. He rejects any notion that human beings are co-creators with God. Nevertheless, he recognizes work as essential to humanity. Work is necessary and meaningful as service in the Kingdom of God. It is done to the glory of God in response to the creative and ruling work of God. Human activity is essentially and optimally cooperation in the ministry of the Christian community, as it witnesses to and proclaims the reality of God's activity. As necessary as work is, it is not an end in itself, nor is it a continuation of the work of God. It is merely obedience to the divine command and fulfillment of natural law. In other words, work attempts to secure survival, prolong life, and earn daily bread so that people can serve the goal of human existence, namely, the Kingdom of God (Barth, 1961).

There are limitations to the kinds of human activity that constitute legitimate work. Only work that fosters the continuation of human existence qualifies. Barth proposes five criteria by which to determine genuine work. The first criterion—what Barth calls *objectivity*—is an end that is consistent with the preservation of human life. A second criterion is the worth of work. Any work that serves the end of preserving human existence intrinsically has worth. For Barth, much modern work is suspect in light of this criterion. The humanity of work is a third criterion. In God's creative intent, work is cooperative coexistence that enables people to participate in the service of the community of faith. A major problem with much modern work is that it is highly individualistic and largely ignores the needs of other people. Because work is social by nature, it necessitates both a recognition of and concern for the needs of others. Much contemporary work, however, is a competitive struggle in which each person strives to live better than others. Thus it largely ignores the cooperative dimension that is essential to truly human work. A fourth criterion of legitimate work is *reflectivity;* that is, inward subjectivity that affirms human existence. The final criterion is *limitation*—the recognition that work is secondary and not all-consuming in human living (Barth, 1961).

Envisioning work as a necessity, Barth makes a fundamental distinction between work as ensuring human survival and the purpose of human existence as service in the Christian community. Because the Kingdom of God is exclusively God's work, people have no part in it at all other than witnessing its reality. Human work, therefore, has no ultimate significance and must not be taken too seriously. Such an outlook provides a sanguine and realistic framework for confronting some of the key issues prevalent in modern work, such as meaninglessness, injustice, and lack of purpose. Barth articulates cogent, insightful, and highly relevant observations and critiques of modern work. His theological assessment of work has the further advantage of not raising high expectations for work. Accordingly, work has its place in life and is to be taken seriously, but it is not the primary dimension of life and must not be taken *too* seriously. The full meaning of human existence is neither exhausted in work nor fully experienced there.

THE GOODNESS OF WORK

Closely allied with the interpretation of work as necessary is the idea that work is intrinsically good. Many biblical writers, for example, affirm the activity of God in the world of work. As Minear (1954, p. 33) points out, the Bible is a "book by workers, about workers, for workers." Minear interprets the biblical perspective as including an integration between specific daily work, the work of others, the whole human experience, and the ultimate divine purposes for human destiny. Such connectedness gives work its true significance (Minear, 1954). In a similar fashion, Barth (1961) sees the essence of human activity, even in work, as movement toward wholeness. A major biblical emphasis is upon the person of the worker and individual motivations for working, rather than upon the specific form work assumes in daily life. Through work, people express something of their inner being, so that work assumes meaning depending upon a person's sense of purpose in life. Hence virtually every occupation is potentially meaningful and receptive to the presence and purpose of God. Because God is the source of human skill and natural resources, the work of God precedes all human work, and divine activity continues alongside human work either to bless or condemn it (Minear, 1954). Divine blessing is essential for human work to be fruitful. In this theological perspective, little credit goes to human effort, because the good results of human labor are the gift of God, who blesses all honest and worthwhile work (Richardson, 1952). As the psalmist poignantly reminds us,

> Unless the Lord builds the house,
> those who build it labor in vain. . . .
> It is in vain that you rise up early and go late to rest,
> eating the bread of anxious toil,
> for he gives sleep to his beloved.
>   (Psalm 127:1a, 2, NRSV)

Intimately related to the meaning of life, work is an essential part of being human. It is also part of God's creative will, not primarily punishment for sin, because even before the Fall, people were given work (see Genesis 1:28; 2:15). Although essentially a blessing, work has been tarnished by human sinfulness and has become a vehicle for self-seeking, conflict, and competiton. The divine curse upon work (see Genesis 3:17–19), moreover, is all too evident in human experience (Richardson,

1952; Minear, 1954). In Genesis 3, God curses not work per se but the soil. Thus it does not necessarily follow that all human work is thereby under a divine curse, although such a view has been traditional in much Christian theology.

In the history of Christian thought, a number of prominent theologians have espoused an interpretation of work as essentially good. In the fifth century, Augustine concluded that work that is aimed at truth, justice, peace, and the social welfare can be a manifestation of divine activity in human history. At the same time, he recognized that self-centered work was ultimately destructive. After the fall of Rome and the emergence of monasticism in the West, Benedict introduced a monastic discipline that included seven hours of manual labor every day except Sunday. Work received new meaning and dignity through the Benedictine influence. By the thirteenth century, Thomas Aquinas recognized work as the primary activity in human civilization. In a hierarchical ordering of both society and church, Aquinas held a high evaluation of all work as contributing to the social order wherein each person did work consistent with his or her abilities, training, and interests (Calhoun, 1954).

In contemporary theology, one of the clearest statements of work as essentially good is the papal encyclical on work issued by John Paul II. The encyclical not only affirms the human dignity of the worker but also postulates that no socioeconomic system can legitimately destroy such dignity. Work is intrinsic to humanity created in the image of God, because it is through work that people realize their basic humanity. Thus work is both a basic human need and a right. The worth and dignity of work correlates with the person of the worker, not with the form of the work nor with the resulting product (Soelle & Cloyes, 1984; Raines & Day-Lower, 1986). The following statement from the encyclical clearly expresses the basic goodness of work: "Work is a great good for man—a good thing for his humanity, because through work man *not only transforms nature*, adapting it to his own needs, but also *achieves fulfillment* as a human being and indeed, in a sense, becomes 'more a human being'" (Raines & Day-Lower, 1986, p. 122).

In a view of work as basically good, the primary motivation for working is gratitude to God. Work is a response to what God has already done for people in Christ. The very fact that the Incarnation came in the form of a village carpenter is for some biblical interpreters a clear affirmation of the worth of human labor. Even though the workplace also manifests hardship, injustice, and drudgery, a Christian views work as redeemed by Christ. Nevertheless, human destiny is broader than work and the ultimate end of life is knowledge and enjoyment of God (Richardson, 1952).

WORK AS VOCATION

A third theological interpretation posits work as an expression of Christian vocation. This view has been most forcefully articulated by the Reformers, especially Martin Luther. Numerous contemporary biblical scholars argue that in applying the concept of "calling" to everyday life, the Reformers expanded biblical perspectives, because there is no explicit biblical reference to a person's being called to an earthly occupation (Richardson, 1952; Calhoun, 1954). Luther based his understanding of vocation on a single verse in the Pauline epistles that is unique in the New Testament in its use of the concept of "calling" (Calhoun, 1954, pp. 88–89; Wingren, 1957, pp. 1–2). "Let each of you remain in the condition in which you were called" (1 Corinthians 7:20, NRSV). Luther interpeted this verse to mean that the call of the gospel comes to Christians in their worldly stations. The call does not necessarily entail a change in occupation or office, because faith and love, which are primary, can be expressed through a variety of occupations, all of which are suitable for people of faith. The individual has little choice about what to do in life but merely accepts his or her given vocation and learns to be content therein.

For Luther, the essence of vocation is love and service of the neighbor in all of life's stations and relationships. The work a person performs in a specific station is obedience to God in the form of serving one's neighbor. God gives each person the work she or he is to do through stations. Neither the Bible nor Christian teaching gets very specific beyond the stipulation that all stations fall within the "common order" of love of God and neighbor. Luther further claimed that the creative work of God continues through human expressions of vocation. In fact, work is one of the "masks" through which God gives people what they need in life, confers blessing on them, and expresses love to them. Human beings function as co-workers with God through their work and prayer; vocation, as Luther interpreted it, actually mediates the divine presence to humanity (Wingren, 1957; Althaus, 1972).

Living out a sense of vocation entails a sensitivity to the present moment combined with an ability to accept life as God gives it. Luther had a keen appreciation for time as not being subject to human manipulation. Because every human work has its proper time to begin and reach fulfillment, no one knows in advance when the proper time will be. Consequently, there is no point in worrying about the future or spending much time planning for it. The life of faith recognizes instead that human beings do not control events but constantly face uncertainty (Althaus, 1972). A contemporary interpreter of vocation, Minear, adds to Luther's position the emphasis that vocation is not something one creates on one's own but is instead a response to a stimulus originating outside oneself. It also provides a pattern of continuity throughout a person's lifetime and contributes significantly to a person's wholeness (Minear, 1977).

Minear identifies in the Old Testament a corporate view of Israel's vocation, which was the context for each person's vocation within the Israelite community. The biblical meaning of vocation thus integrates the life and work of individuals with that of the wider community, so that every type of work contributes to Israel's corporate vocation. The central reality in biblical vocation is always the God who calls people to a purpose. In the New Testament, moreover, every job is a form of service to God, and every human activity is a response to the call of God. Vocation represents, therefore, the intersection between divine and human work. The realization of the Kingdom of God will confirm the validity of Christian vocation in contradistinction to worldly standards of power, success, status, and ambition. Until then, Christ is the norm of vocation inasmuch as he inaugurates the restoration of the original human vocation (Minear, 1977).

An understanding of work as vocation, epitomized in the thought of Luther and Minear, has much to say to the contemporary workplace. It implies that people of faith share a common vocation, yet each individual has a special work to perform. If work is not a vehicle for vocation in this sense, it is without meaning or worth.

WORK AS CO-CREATION

A fourth and somewhat controversial typology is work as co-creation, as found in the thought of futurist Barbara Marx Hubbard and theologian Dorothee Soelle, both of whom claim that human energy and activity enjoy a partnership with God. Soelle is highly critical of the radical distinction traditional Christian theology makes between God the Creator and human beings as creatures. She regards an absolutely transcendent God as an independent male figure completely separate from created reality in contradistinction to God as interdependent and interrelated with creation and humanity. If the divine-human relationship is reciprocal, vocation values human creativity in relation to both God and others, so that people are affirmed as co-creators with God in the work of love and justice (Soelle, 1984). For Soelle, human creativity is the ability "to renew the world for someone or for a community," and creation is "an opening process" that remains unfinished (Soelle, 1984, p. 37). The human worker is a living expression of ongoing creation. Her view does not, however, diminish the work of God, for as Soelle explains, "The more a person develops her creativity, delves into the project of liberation, and transcends her own limitations, the more God is God" (p. 39).

Soelle identifies three fundamental dimensions of work: self-expression, relatedness to society, and reconciliation with nature. The practical conclusions she draws are strikingly similar to Barth's criteria for genuine work. In the first dimension of self-expression, Soelle argues that meaningful, fulfilling work is a basic human need and necessary for full human development. The subjective aspect of good work includes both self-realization and dignity. In the second dimension of social relatedness, the essentially cooperative character of work is affirmed in a recognition that truly good work entails a relinquishing of egocentricity. When that occurs, the "divine self" within each person can be expressed as service to others through human cooperation. Finally, the dimension of reconciliation with nature anticipates the realization of a humane new world through the fruits of human labor, in contrast to the exploitation and destruction of nature that is the tragic but unnecessary consequence of much modern technology.

Although Soelle constructs her theology of co-creation upon an interpretation of Genesis 1:27–28, where humanity is given dominion over creation, other theologians, notably Barth and Richardson, make a radical distinction between creativity—which they attribute exclusively to God—and human dominion over creation. Whereas Soelle presents God as "power-in-relationship" and humanity as participating in the ongoing creative work of God, Richardson claims that in the Bible human work is never creative in the same sense as divine activity. Through their dominion over creation, people share in God's lordship but not in divine creativity. Furthermore, the general usage of the term *work* in the Bible implies routine, boring labor that is neither creative nor goal oriented. One of the reasons human work is not portrayed more significantly in the Bible is the Hebrew aversion to idolatry—a further matter that now requires our attention (Richardson, 1952).

WORK AS IDOLATRY

None of the theological typologies we have examined thus far has any sympathy for an idolatrous view of work, in which human activity in effect is substituted for the creative work of God. Biblical writers avoided exalting human labor for fear that it would become idolatrous. Barth (1961), for one, interprets human culture as the highest form of work with the greatest potential for obscuring the divine reality, if it is not recognized as the limited and creaturely activity it is. Soelle (1984, p. 109) even goes so far as to assert that modern technology has supplanted the God of creation and become "the new demon." An idolatrous view makes work the obsession of human existence and attributes ultimate qualities to human products with the result that people live solely in a "human-made" world. Arendt (1958) recognizes the tendency toward such idolatry in her eloquent depiction of "human artifice" as the subjection of nature to human influence and the replacement of biological subjectivity with human-made objectivity. When human work so alienates people from participation in natural life rhythms and cycles, the effect is neither salutary nor beneficial. Human ego strives to be independent and bend nature to its desires. Under such circumstances, humanity fails to recognize its participation in nature, its unity with it, its interdependence with other aspects of creation, and its union with the ground of being. A classic example of idolatrous work is the Tower of Babel incident in Genesis 11:1–9, where the prime motivation for the workers is to make a name for themselves. Idolatrous work presumes that through their own efforts people can become self-sufficient. In denying an interrelatedness with all things in the universe, humanity can potentially usurp the creative activity of God. Two other biblical passages that strongly condemn the worship of human fabrications are Psalm 115:2–4ff. and Isaiah 44:9–20. Although modern workers do not engage in the precise forms of idolatry described in such passages, many do place their ultimate trust in human works, such as technology, science, and medicine. All such attitudes are tantamount to a new form of idolatry in which human work becomes a total preoccupation to the exclusion of the divine reality.

COMMON THEMES AND APPLICATIONS

Even though there are different assessments of the meaning of work among the four typologies we have thus far examined, some common conclusions offer important insights for the modern workplace. The theologians cited agree that most modern work is dehumanizing and does not conform to the will and purpose of God. In spite of its perversions, they see work as God given, necessary, purposeful, and valuable. Furthermore most theologians define work as cooperative activity intended to serve others, rather than individualistic ego-centrism.[1]

A fourth point of convergence is the role of rest and leisure as a counterbalance to work. Martin Luther claimed that when people rest, they worship God most completely, because that is when they place their trust most radically in God (Althaus, 1972). His insight is very apropos for modern American culture, where so much of a person's life is centered around work. Technology is making possible a shorter work week, medicine is lengthening life spans, and more and more people can anticipate a significant period of retirement in good health. As a result, a theological perspective on leisure and recreation is a necessary corollary of a theology of work (Nelson, 1954).

From a purely human perspective, people can contribute to society with their work. At the same time, the world does not fall apart whenever people stop working to rest, because God as Creator continues to preserve life. In similar fashion, Barth argues that secular work is not the ultimate meaning of human activity and therefore needs to be balanced and properly limited with rest. In part, this means that people work under orders from a superior and are neither able nor expected to complete the divine creative purpose through their labor. God has already done it for humanity. Compulsive work therefore denies the lordship of God as the one in charge of creation (Barth, 1961).

In the biblical tradition, observance of the Sabbath acknowledged that work was not the dominant goal nor the most important activity in life. Instead life consists of a rhythm between work and rest with a clear delineation between the two. Rest does not connote idleness, as modern people are prone to think, but a dynamic experience that includes worship. Sabbath rest anticipates eschatological rest in the Kingdom of God. Because earthly work is merely transitory and ephemeral, it does not become the primary source of significance for human existence. What gives work lasting meaning and value is its anticipated fulfillment in the Kingdom of God (Richardson, 1952). In sum, it is possible and even desirable to take human work seriously, yet not *too* seriously. A healthy pattern of rest and leisure contributes to a balanced perspective that avoids the perversity of work as idolatry. Human confidence in the incessant work of God frees people for rest and leisure in the assurance that they do not have to do everything themselves. As Luther recognized before the advent of modern industrialism, people can relax without being anxious, because the fate of the universe does not depend on them.

APPLICATIONS TO THE WORKPLACE

Beyond the unifying themes among the various typologies of work, a number of other applications to the workplace emanate from a theological perspective. I will now set forth some of my own views on the theology of work in dialogue with the positions summarized in preceding sections.

The Conceptualization of Work

An apparent difficulty in much theological reflection is a rather narrow conception of work as a job or a remunerated activity performed in order to provide for basic life needs. I see a need for a more comprehensive understanding of work. Many people do significant work without remuneration. A more comprehensive conception of work would encompass people not usually considered—homemakers, volunteers, retired people, the disabled, the handicapped, the unemployed, and so on. Capra, a physicist, has recently advocated on secular grounds a major redefinition of work. He points out that two-thirds of all wages paid in the United States is the monetary equivalent of the noncompensated work in households alone (Capra, 1982).

Some theologians have attempted a broader conceptualization of work. Soelle, for example, rejects the identification of work with compensated activity and proposes that work can be meaningful in itself (Soelle, 1984). Minear also envisions a more comprehensive definition of work that recognizes its systemic character whereby all parts of an economic system are interconnected, affect the whole, and are in turn affected by the whole. For him, work is a much broader phenomenon than activity performed to secure basic life necessities: "that universal, agelong activity of man by which he seeks to sustain, to vindicate, to realize that which as man he seeks in life" (Minear, 1954, p. 37). Some such systemic view of work as contributing the conditions necessary for humane existence can be an invaluable perspective in the workplace. Raines and Day-Lower in their recent study of work in America have formulated an understanding of work as "the direct expression of a unique human excellence, a direct expression of the way we humans establish ourselves in this world, develop ourselves, and in a sense perfect ourselves as a species." For them, work is a uniquely human way of both "being and becoming" (Raines & Day-Lower, 1986, pp. 14–15).

The term *lifework* is one way of expressing a broader concept of work, especially if it includes any human activity that gives meaning, purpose, and direction to life. It is possibly a generic concept for thinking theologically about work. As I read and interpret the New Testament, I see that Jesus had a sense of mission in life that he had been given by God. In John 5:17, for example, he refers to his own activity and that of God as *work*. Again in John 9:4, he characterizes his messianic ministry as work with a metaphor drawn from everyday work. (For other descriptions of Jesus's ministry as the work of one who had sent him, see John 4:34 and 17:4.) Jesus's mission expressed through his earthly ministry, not his work as a carpenter, was really his lifework, as I am using the term here. Similarly, even though St. Paul was a tent maker by trade (Acts 18:3; 1 Corinthians 4:12), he saw his ministry to the Gentiles as at least analogous to work. In 1 Corinthians 3:5–15, Paul uses metaphors from manual labor (agriculture and construction) for his ministry. He even refers at one point to the Corinthian church as "God's farm, God's building." There is a biblical basis, therefore, for conceiving of work as that which people do out of a sense of calling that gives their lives meaning, direction, and purpose.

A major difficulty in the modern American workplace is that few jobs and occupations offer people much meaning. People want meaning, but few are finding it in their jobs. Thus there remain some perplexing questions in the workplace. Is it possible, or even appropriate, to expect meaning in work? Is it realistic for people to search for work that offers a sense of worth, satisfaction, and purpose? If not, where might meaning in life be found? I will return to such questions shortly. A broader conceptualization of work as purposive lifework or human being/becoming provides a fruitful context for discerning meaning that is not possible when work is limited to gainful employment. From a Christian perspective, it is also impossible to comprehend mission or purpose in life apart from a vision of the divine creative purpose that will be fully realized only in the Kingdom of God.

The Transformation of Work in Modern Society

The current upheaval in forms of employment has serious repercussions for future understandings of work. The shift that is presently occurring from an industrial era to one centered around service and information is as extensive as earlier shifts from an agricultural to an industrial economy. Unfortunately, much of the theological critique of work is concerned with the lamentable impact of industrialization upon human work.

The study by Raines and Day-Lower graphically substantiates the painful displacement and personally devastating effects of the disintegration of jobs, culture, and a social system generated by an industrial economy. Although Raines and Day-Lower recognize that American society is experiencing rapid and extensive upheaval in the workplace, their prognosis for the short term at least is that most workers displaced by unemployment and underemployment will have a lower standard of living, even if they find new forms of work. Their view is a fairly pessimistic one for the immediately foreseeable future (Raines & Day-Lower, 1986). The impressive evidence amassed in their study documents the painful realities and the ensuing dissipation during the transition from an industrial to a post-industrial economy.

In short, the world of work is undergoing dramatic change. Many of the people now being forced into the ranks of the unemployed by developments such as automation and robotics are least equipped to adapt to the changing work environment. Similar dissipations have characterized previous transformations in human history, but in no instance has the disruption and the endemic human suffering been the final word. Humanity has weathered each crisis and moved on to new forms of social and economic organization. Few people today would seriously consider returning to the medieval feudal system of Luther's time. Change in any sector of life is difficult and can be tragic, but not all upheaval is negative. In the long run, the consequences of an epochal transition may well be quite beneficial.

In light of the contemporary transformation in work, how can we reflect theologically about a phenomenon that continues to change as we contemplate it? What if the forms of work that are now emerging in post-industrial society are merely a temporary phase in the further evolution and development of work? Theology needs to think and talk about work in a way that encompasses emerging new realities. It is highly probable that in the next twenty-five years work will undergo even more radical changes than we have encountered to date. Neither theology nor career theory has adequately articulated principles that illuminate and elucidate the new social, economic, and cultural phenomena that are already operative in the workplace, to say nothing of those that are likely to characterize the workplace in the future. The perspective on the social order reflected both in the biblical writers and in Martin Luther—fruitful sources for a theology of work—is hierarchical and static. The outlook of modern science and much of contemporary society, by contrast, recognizes change as the constant and perceives reality as essentially flow, movement, and process.[2]

In thinking theologically about work, therefore, does one begin with a static hierarchical view of the social order with God as the source of that order? Or can one begin with a dynamic view of the social order in which God is the power within, behind, and beyond the flux that moves the whole process through meaningful patterns and realizes purpose through the vagaries of change? What would be the theological and practical effects of detaching an understanding of vocation from fixed social stations and applying it to a complex social matrix of ever-changing roles and relationships?

The process theology Soelle uses in her reflections on work has potential for interpeting the profound breakthroughs and reconceptualizations of reality introduced into modern consciousness through science. In such a theology, becoming and dynamic relationship take precedence over being and hierarchy. God always possesses potential beyond what has been expressed in the past and the present and continually offers humanity new possibilities without predetermining what people will choose (Soelle, 1984). With a theological vision of divine activity in and through dramatic changes in the human experience, it may be possible to affirm some hopeful patterns and potentialities in the confusion besetting the workplace. The radical upheavals we are now experiencing may themselves be hopeful signs. The industrial system that is being replaced produced many forms of everyday work that to a large degree have frustrated and bored modern workers, even to the point of seriously eroding their human dignity. The loss of such a system that often stultifies and represses human potential may well be a long-term gain. At least it offers the possibility that work can and will be vastly different. Soelle (1984) also suggests that even unemployment can be an opportunity to reconceptualize work in ways that restore satisfaction and dignity and reaffirm human interdependence.

One implication of a society characterized by increased leisure, yet one in which people have basic life necessities, is that people may be able to choose meaningful activities without concern for compensation. A good example is the situation of E., described at the beginning of this chapter. In many ways in the prime of her life with a support system secured, she is free to pursue whatever may give her life meaning and purpose. During the last twenty-five years, I have encountered numerous people with similar economic and occupational possibilities—government employees, career military personnel, police, successful entrepreneurs, to mention only a few. There is no assurance such people will perceive or take advantage of the manifold opportunities available. Even so, I am convinced there is much potential good in the upheaval we are undergoing. I am even more firmly convinced we need a theological vision capable of illuminating our present confusion and giving people hope and confidence by pointing a meaningful direction toward future fulfillment.

The Recovery of Meaning
Through a Sense of Vocation

The Christian concept of vocation speaks directly to the seminal issue of meaning in work and offers the possibility of transforming human attitudes about work. Raines and Day-Lower (1986) argue that a much-needed theological articulation of work can be discovered through a revival of the concept of vocation. They further contend that a theology of work must address the critical question of the meaning of work. I strongly concur with both suggestions. As previously intimated, vocation is a concept broad enough to encompass an expanded definition of work, because it is not limited to compensated employment. Ideally, people of faith bring a sense of vocation to their employment, whatever it may be, and concentrate their time and energy upon finding appropriate ways to live and work meaningfully and purposefully. Work does not have to be devoid of either meaning or purpose, yet neither are automatic concomitants of work. A strong sense of vocation grounded in faith makes possible the apprehension and expression of meaning in life and work.

Ephesians 4:1–6 provides a comprehensive vision of vocation that is grounded in unity and fullness:

> I, therefore, the prisoner in the Lord, beg you to lead a life worthy of the calling to which you have been called, with all humility and gentleness, with patience, bearing with one another in love, making every effort to maintain the unity of the Spirit in the bond of peace. There is one body and one Spirit, just as you were called to the one hope of your calling, one Lord, one faith, one baptism, one God and Father of all, who is above all and through all and in all. (NRSV)

Even though this passage is primarily depicting the mystical Body of Christ, if the work of Christ and the mission of the mystical Body affirm the world/cosmos as the primary domain of divine activity, it does not seem unreasonable to expect that growth in Christ can and should occur in all aspects of life and human relationships.

The Ephesians passage also recognizes that each individual, as part of a larger unity, has a specific function to fulfill within that unity. Raines and Day-Lower (1986) in particular are concerned about the excessive individualism that characterizes the American orientation to work. They detect an alienation between individual work and the common good, as well as a loss of a sense of interdependence through work. They further suggest that a sense of vocation can restore the all-important communal dimension of human work.

Other observers of the American workplace have also identified excessive individualism as a major component in the erosion of meaning in work. One recent, well-publicized sociological analysis of American culture laments the loss of a sense of "calling" in work whereby individuals relate to others and the wider society through their work. Such work can be intrinsically meaningful and valuable in the context of human community (Bellah, Madsen, Sullivan, Swidler, & Tipton, 1985). Similarly, Studs Terkel in his encyclopedic survey of work in America quotes Nora Watson: "I think most of us are looking for a calling, not a job. Most of us . . . have jobs that are too small for our spirit" (Terkel, 1972, p. xxiv).

The corporate understanding of vocation, already identified in the Old Testament view of the vocation of Israel, is a significant corrective to the excessive individualism that predominates in modern America. A theology of vocation relates work first and foremost to the common good, rather than to individual benefit. All Christians have a common calling to serve God and neighbor, but each individual in turn matches his or her gifts with particular needs and tasks in the human community (Raines & Day-Lower, 1986). Buechner (1993) has succinctly captured a communal orientation by claiming that true vocation emerges where a person's gifts and natural interests coincide with a real need in the world.

Biblical writers, especially in the New Testament, were preoccupied with the spread of the gospel under conditions of persecution and duress, as well as with the imminence of the *eschaton* (the end of history). They attributed only limited theological significance to secular work and did not concern themselves very much with the implications of the gospel for the workplace (Richardson, 1952). The Bible, as the norm and rule of Christian faith, does not speak extensively to contemporary work experience. A question thus remains as to how Christians are to view work and interpret its meaning. Raines and Day-Lower (1986) respond that meaning is a fundamental human need; therefore people need to understand the meaning of what they do in work. In fact, the primary way people participate in society and gain a feeling of making a contribution to others is through work.

I would add that in modern America secular work is also a prime context for Christian witness—a witness that may never be heeded if it is confined to the institutional church. The Reformation, in my view, properly broadened the New Testament understanding of Christian vocation to everyday work and social stations (Richardson, 1952), but it did so within a static conception of a hierarchical social order. What happens to the traditional Reformation emphasis on vocation if work is seen as a dynamic phenomenon in a rapidly changing social milieu? I would affirm with Luther that all Christians share a common vocation, which can be expressed through many different roles, relationships, and occupations, and I would agree with Raines and Day-Lower that the concept of vocation applies to people in all forms of work. Unlike Luther, however, I would contend that people are not limited to the social stations or occupations in which they find themselves. In endeavoring to be a faithful steward of one's God-given gifts and abilities, a Christian seeks the fullest expression of personhood in the service of God and neighbor. Through work, people come to understand and experience human history as purposeful, insofar as they participate in historical evolution and contribute to it through their work (Minear, 1954). Unless this is the case, people cannot realize or even approximate their human potential. In the contemporary workplace, vocation is an ever-unfolding sensitivity to meaning and purpose in life that can be neither exhausted nor depleted by any single role or by any number of roles or occupations in the life span of an individual. Vocation as a theological concept applied to the world of work is virtually unlimited in its applications and implications. As Minear (1954) aptly points out, vocation concentrates on the comprehension of life purpose through a combination of divine revelation and voluntary human obedience. Human existence is thus a lifelong discovery of the implications of vocation in all aspects of life, including work, for both the individual Christian and the community of faith.

CONCLUSION

I began with several examples of people who were struggling with the question of meaning in their work. I have now come full circle to argue that the Christian idea of vocation affords people today a significant way to discover and affirm meaning in their work. I have been privileged to know many people whose lives are informed by a sense of vocation, but one of the best examples is a person I encountered in a career planning workshop. M. is a happily married woman in her early fifties employed part-time as a registered nurse in an institution for the elderly. When asked about her work, she quickly replies that she loves it and cannot imagine herself doing anything other than nursing in some form, albeit not necessarily with the elderly or in her present job. The key for her is responding concretely to human needs in a loving and compassionate manner. Even in her personal life apart from her job, she enjoys visiting with elderly people in her neighborhood and responding directly to their needs with simple acts of service. During the summer, she works as a nurse at a church camp, where her favorite people are mentally challenged campers. When she describes what these people have meant to her, tears come into her eyes. A number of them, I have since learned, regard M. as one of their best friends. Although M. would probably not articulate her sense of meaning in life in terms of vocation, she is a living example of a person who blends faith and work with motivation, a sense of purpose, and an orientation to others and their needs that is the essence of vocation.

Theology, or "God-talk," can speak to the contemporary workplace. In fact, it has an important message for workers. Its message is that work can and should be meaningful and that people have a right to find meaning in work. The route to the discovery of meaning in work is a responsive awareness of both God and neighbor that takes seriously the resources people have been given, needs in society and the wider world, and the will of God as apprehended by faith.

NOTES

1. Barth, pp. 474–478, especially articulates the conclusions epitomized in this paragraph.
2. For a comprehensive and highly readable interpretation of the views of modern physics, see Capra, F., *The tao of physics*. New York: Bantam Books.

REFERENCES

Althaus, P. (1972). *The ethics of Martin Luther.* Philadelphia: Fortress Press.

Arendt, H. (1958). *The human condition*. Chicago: University of Chicago Press.

Barth, K. (1961). *Church dogmatics, III,* Part 4. Edinburgh: T&T Clark.

Bellah, R. N., Madsen, R., Sullivan, W. M., Swidler, A., & Tipton, S. M. (1985). *Habits of the heart: Individualism and commitment in American life*. Berkeley: University of California Press.

Buechner, F. (1993). *Wishful thinking*. San Francisco: Harper San Francisco.

Calhoun, R. (1954). Work and vocation in Christian history. In J. O. Nelson (Ed.), *Work and vocation*. New York: HarperCollins.

Capra, F. (1982). *The turning point*. Toronto, Ont.: Bantam Books.

Minear, P. (1977). *To die and to live: Christ's resurrection and Christian vocation*. New York: Seabury.

Minear, P. (1954). Work and vocation in scripture. In J. O. Nelson (Ed.), *Work and vocation*. New York: HarperCollins.

Nelson, J. O. (1954) Introduction. In J. O. Nelson (Ed.), *Work and vocation: A Christian discussion*. New York: HarperCollins.

Raines, J. C., & Day-Lower, D. C. (1986). *Modern work and human meaning.*
Philadelphia: Westminster Press.
Richardson, A. (1952). *The biblical doctrine of work.* London: SCM Press.
Soelle, D., with Cloyes, S. A. (1984). *To work and to love: A theology of creation.*
Philadelphia: Fortress.
Terkel, S. (1972). *Working.* New York: Pantheon.
Wingren, G. (1957). *Luther on vocation.* Philadelphia: Muhlenberg Press.

PART TWO

APPLICATIONS: CONNECTING SPIRIT AND CAREER

CHAPTER SEVEN

Creating Personal and Spiritual Balance

Another Dimension in Career Development

Marian Stoltz-Loike
Windham International

Spirituality is not often a component of the discussion in the career development literature on balancing work and personal concerns. Typically the discussion focuses on gender differences in career concerns (e.g., Gati, Osipow, & Givon, 1995; Rowe & Snizek, 1995), or the conflict between work and family issues (e.g., Mackey, 1995), or the spillover that occurs between disparate aspects of one's life (e.g., Hyde, Klein, Essex, & Clark, 1995). Developing one's spiritual self takes an initial investment of time and energy and an ongoing time commitment to continue that development. When work is all-consuming there is clearly little time for anything else, whether those other aspects involve relationships, family, leisure, or spirituality.

My personal belief is that the ways in which people build relationships, interact with family and friends, and structure their leisure time are all manifestations of their spiritual life. Devoting time to spiritual growth can lead to better balance in life roles and thereby result in more creative development in other aspects of life. Choices are constantly being made about how to behave toward other people, whether precedence is given to work, personal, or family concerns, or to how structured or unstructured leisure time may be. Each of these choices becomes woven together into a tapestry that reflects our past and becomes the prologue to the next chapter of our lives.

In this chapter, I will review the literature on work-family concerns that address the issue of balance. Next I will discuss some of the gender development literature that differentially identifies how men and women create meaning in their lives. Finally, I will speak from a personal perspective about how I have tried to create balance in my own life to allow my spirituality to develop and permeate all aspects of my life.

WORK-FAMILY CONCERNS

Research on work-family concerns in the 1990s has moved beyond those studies that unsuccessfully looked for a variety of negative outcomes in families where mothers were employed (e.g., Bronfenbrenner & Crouter, 1982; Cotton, Antill, & Cunningham, 1990; Greenberger, Goldberg, Crawford, & Granger, 1988; Hiller & Dyehouse, 1987; Hiller & Philliber, 1986; Hoffman & Nye, 1974; Philliber & Hiller, 1978). Instead, recent research has focused on issues within the couple that may affect child development (e.g., Hyde, Klein, Essex, & Clark, 1995) or marital satisfaction (e.g., Rushing & Schwabe, 1995), influence general concerns about family well-being (e.g., Brintnell, Madill, Montgomerie, & Stewin, 1992), or lead to spillover between work and family issues (Hughes & Galinsky, 1994; Kirchmeyer, 1993; Sears & Galambos, 1992; Williams & Alliger, 1994).

With more than 60 percent of women in the labor force, female employment has become the norm for American women. However, women still tend to have more responsibility for housework (Napholz, 1995; Stohs, 1995; Zhang & Farley, 1995), have more discontinuous employment than men (Duncan, Prus, & Sandy, 1993; Felmlee, 1995; Schneer & Reitman, 1995; Stohs, 1992; Voydanoff, 1988), are more likely to be employed part-time (Schneer & Reitman, 1995), and may have different patterns of job involvement than men (Duncan, Prus, & Sandy, 1993; Joesch, 1994; Potuchek, 1992).

Definition of Success

When reflecting on their lives, men and women use different criteria for evaluating success and giving priority to work or family issues (Williams,

1990). Women consider both career and relationship issues (Horst, 1995), whereas men predominantly focus on career issues (Silverman, 1995; Spiker-Miller & Kees, 1995), meaning that women are more vulnerable to spillover effects between work and personal issues (Barnett, Raudenbush, Brennan, Pleck, & Marshall, 1995).

Light (1984) found that women who reported having greater commitment to their careers than their families had significantly higher anxiety than women who reportedly placed greater priority on their families. Moreover, women who reported equal commitments to work and family concerns experienced the greatest degree of work-family conflict, and greater levels of depression, lower self-esteem, and lower life satisfaction (Lobel, 1991). Napholz (1995) also found that women who attributed greater importance to relationships than to work expressed the fewest role conflicts, whereas women who placed priority on work over relationships or valued work and relationships equally had significantly higher levels of depression.

Household Division of Labor

Women still have greater responsibility for household labor (Coverman & Sheley, 1986; Loscocco & Roschelle, 1991; Napholz, 1995; Stohs, 1995; Thompson & Walker, 1989; Zhang & Farley, 1995). The extent of that discrepancy is difficult to determine because some studies evaluate the difference in terms of absolute number of hours each partner is engaged in housework, whereas other studies look at the relative involvement of the two partners. What is clear is that women engage in substantially more hours of housework than men do, probably about ten to twelve hours more per week (Berardo, Shehan, & Leslie, 1987; Stohs, 1995) and in different types of household tasks (Beckwith, 1992). Although studies have shown an inverse relationship between women's earnings and the time they spend in household tasks (Blair & Johnson, 1992), even professional women tend to have more domestic responsibilities than their partners (Tesch, Osborne, Simpson, Murray, & Spiro, 1992). Differences in household division of labor are robust and have been replicated in a variety of cross-cultural settings (Beckwith, 1992; Nakhaie, 1995; Nettles, 1995). Barnett, Raudenbush, Brennan, Pleck, and Marshall (1995) underscore the curiosity of this finding. They argue that because a majority of women in the United States are employed, employment is a central component of the adult lives of men and women. The fact that women as well as men still hold females responsible for family well-being demonstrates that the change in expectations about partner roles is not parallel to the changes evident in employment roles.

Men and women's satisfaction with the division of labor is related to their gender role beliefs (McHale & Crouter, 1992; Pina & Bengsten, 1993) and the different views they hold about the equitable balance of household tasks (Benin & Agostinelli, 1988; Danser & Gilbert, 1993; Yogev & Brett, 1985). Men feel that housework division is fairly balanced when their responsibilities do not take too long to complete, whereas women feel that the division is fair when men take on those jobs that are stereotyped as women's responsibilities (Benin & Agostinelli, 1988; Blair & Johnson, 1992).

Work-Family Conflict

In a comprehensive review of the literature on job satisfaction, Hanson and Sloane (1992) found no relation between job satisfaction among men or women and the presence of young children in the home. Contrary to intuitive expectations, this finding means that whereas the presence of pre-schoolers may make parental roles more complex, they do not make them less satisfying.

Both men and women experience conflict when they balance multiple roles (e.g., Bird & Ford, 1985; Loerch, Russell, & Rush, 1989; Tiedje, et al., 1990). Yet women experience greater role strain from the child-related variables than men do even when there is an equitable division of labor (Bird & Ford, 1985). Part-time employed women seem to experience more work overload and conflict but also more satisfaction with their jobs, marital life, and parental roles than full-time employed women (Barker, 1993).

Flexibility is one measure of a family's ability to negotiate a balance within the workplace between work and family roles (Stoltz-Loike, 1992). Parents who do not have any flexibility at work are more likely to plan to change employment positions (Rothausen, 1994), whereas parents with greater flexibility are more likely to experience less role strain (Guelzow, Bird, & Koball, 1991). Furthermore, parents who feel they have more control over their work environments are likely to experience less work-family conflict (Voydanoff, 1988).

Involvement in housework and other work and parental roles influences the ability that people have for engaging in business-related activities such as networking or after-work socializing and also affects their access to discretionary time to develop hobbies, outside interests, or their spiritual sides. Moreover, despite all of the recent innovations in the ways we work, including telecommuting and greater flexibility, that would seem to support family-friendly organizations, the workplace is still structured with the assumption that workers will be physically present (Perlow, 1995). Thus even parents who have primary childcare responsibilities may feel significant pressures to spend more time in the workplace, even if their companies offer options for doing work at home.

Values

A majority of women are employed today, but women's feelings about whether they should be working or home with children affect their satisfaction with their jobs and the stress they experience (Morgan & Hock, 1984; Potuchek, 1992). Women who were career oriented and wanted to be employed reported that they were happier with their lives when they were employed full-time than a comparable group of women who were employed part-time or were unemployed (Pietromonaco, Manis, & Markus, 1987). In contrast, there was no obvious benefit in mental health or self-esteem among women who were not career oriented (Pietromonaco, Manis, & Markus, 1987).

Although the majority of women are employed, their work parameters vary substantially and society still finds multiple career options, including part-time work and unemployment, acceptable for women. In contrast, men are expected to work full-time unless they are in school or on disability leave. I have found virtually no studies exploring stress issues of full-time employment among men who are career oriented or not, nor studies of how men experience part-time employment as an option for balancing work-family issues. Although there may be far fewer men than women working part-time or working as homemakers to balance work-family concerns, men in those family arrangements seem to be more than the "Mr. Mom" curiosities of a decade ago and deserve greater attention in the research literature.

In a recent study, Hyde, Klein, Essex, and Clark (1995) interviewed women at four months postpartum and found that women who were employed part-time or were full-time homemakers experienced less anxiety than full-time workers. Women who were depressed at four months postpartum were more likely to have taken a short maternity leave and have poor-quality marriages, indicating that returning to the workplace was not related to greater depression among mothers unless they also had other risk factors.

Whether or not women experience work and family conflict may be related to whether they are employed full-time or part-time and whether their career history is continuous or discontinuous. Single women seem to work the same number of hours and have the same work patterns, including extended work hours, as single men (Seron & Ferris, 1995). When they evaluate their jobs, men and women both similarly identify (1) feelings of accomplishment, (2) high income, and (3) opportunity for advancement as being more important work values than job security or shorter working hours (Rowe & Snizek, 1995).

Across the studies of the interaction of work and family variables, few studies control for whether the men and women used as subjects in the study are employed full-time or part-time, outside of the home or from within their homes. This is an unfortunate oversight, because factors such as flextime or flex place can be important variables affecting employee attitude toward work, especially in studies of work-family issues (see, for example, Stoltz-Loike, 1992). Rowe and Snizek (1995) indicate that they found few differences between men and women because their subjects were all employed full-time outside of their homes.

Workplace Policy

Balancing work and family issues is of paramount importance to the mental health of men and women (Rushing & Schwabe, 1995) and for the ability of male and female workers to achieve upward mobility (Mackey, 1995). One of the most significant ways that organizations can help parents is by providing family-friendly benefits to employees, which may include flexible benefits, childcare and eldercare, leave policies, and access to Employee Assistance Programs (see Stoltz-Loike, 1992, for a comprehensive review).

Despite the fact that offering family-friendly benefits makes good business sense, many organizations now offer only limited support. Glass and Fujimoto (1995) found that larger organizations were the most likely to offer leaves to their employees, and unionization correlated with higher-quality leave benefits. In contrast, work schedule policies that encourage flexibility are more likely to be offered at the discretion of individual managers. It is no surprise that benefits requiring the greatest degree of supervisor support are more likely to be left to informal personnel management decisions. Summarizing their findings, Glass and Fujimoto (1995) underscore that childcare support is the easiest to provide and the least disruptive to organizational life. Flexible benefits and leave policies provide the child's primary caretaker with the most meaningful support in balancing multiple roles and are also the most challenging to implement.

Conjoint Career Counseling

Career counselors can play significant roles in developing new methods to address work-family concerns. In particular, family systems theory (see review in Stoltz-Loike, 1992) provides a useful starting point for developing new strategies. Family systems theory assumes that families operate like chemical or physical systems. Systems exist in equilibrium. Any time one part of the system is disrupted, it creates turbulence in the rest of the system, which then tries to reestablish equilibrium. Within families, this means that change can only be effective when the whole family evolves simultaneously. Otherwise, other parts of the system (i.e., family members) will oppose any attempt at change undertaken by just one family member.

One of the most productive applications of family systems theory is for dual-career couples in conjoint career counseling (Forrest, 1994; Spiker-Miller & Kees, 1995; Stoltz-Loike, 1992). This approach involves simultaneously providing couples with the opportunity to consider the impact of any career change that one person makes on the partner's career and on the family. Counseling options will vary with the career stage of each partner and the family stage as a couple. Both partners are involved in all sessions in this form of career counseling.

Sekaran (1986) and Hazard and Koslow (1986) have outlined six stages in family development. During counseling, it is assumed that early development affects later stages and that couples need to constantly focus on balancing family and career needs, managing time, providing mutual support, reassessing family stage, and expressing their commitments to the family. The career, personal, and family challenges that people face differ at each stage, as do the appropriate solutions. By considering all of these arenas and including both partners in counseling, counselors can help couples reach the most productive and effective work-family solutions.

GENDER ISSUES

Gender differences have been found throughout the career development arena, beginning with differences in career aspirations among children and teenagers (Farmer, Wardrop, Anderson, & Risinger, 1995; Gassin, Kelly, & Feldhusen, 1993; Levine & Zimmerman, 1995), choice of math and science courses (Sandqvist, 1995), and mathematical self-efficacy (Terwillinger & Titus, 1995).

Within the career development arena, women and men are more likely to choose different career fields in college (Farmer, Wardrop, Anderson, & Risinger, 1995). Female undergraduates have been shown to place more importance on work enjoyment, self-efficacy, and people (Lips, 1992) and to have higher levels of work commitment (Luzzo, 1994). Young men are more likely than women to find a job through a friend, remain in a job longer, use fewer job search strategies with greater success, and have a close relationship with a mentor/supervisor.

These differences have been of some concern to counselors, educators, and public policy makers, because of the discrepancy evident later in life between the career choices that men and women make. Irrespective of early career aspirations, women are still less likely to choose careers in science, math, or technical fields (Farmer, Wardrop, Anderson, & Risinger, 1995; Levine & Zimmerman, 1995). Additionally, in a variety of different fields, women have had greater difficulty in moving up the organizational ladder (Schneer & Reitman, 1995).

Workplace Differences

In their study, Schneer and Reitman (1995) compared the career paths of male and female MBAs. They found that early in their careers, one-fourth of women were not employed full-time, and at mid-career one-fifth of women were not employed full-time. At either point, only a very few men were not employed on a full-time basis. Furthermore, a differential in earnings between men and women appeared shortly after they received their MBAs and rose to 19 percent by seven to twelve years post-MBA. By mid-career, only 9 percent of the women had made it to the executive suite, compared with 25 percent of the men. Despite these differences, women and men were equally satisfied with their careers. In a separate study, men were found to reach middle management positions faster and through fewer promotions than women (Morgan, Schor, & Martin, 1993).

Gender differences also exist with regard to employment positions of men and women. In a study of psychologists, women were more likely to be practitioners, whereas men were more likely to be faculty members (Reschly & Wilson, 1995; Wilson & Reschly, 1995). Male doctors were more likely to show concern with practical and tangible aspects of medical practice, whereas women were more concerned with psychosocial aspects of medical care (Hojat, Gonnella, & Xu, 1995). Among psychologists, men rated prestige and salary as more important than did women, whereas women rated work schedule flexibility as more important than did men (McGowen & Hart, 1992).

Once women and men have entered the job market, they have different market experiences of the workplace. Women earn approximately 64 cents on the dollar compared to what men earn, with the ratio varying between 51 percent and parity (Anderson & Tomaskovic-Devey, 1995). Some of the greatest discrepancies between earnings of men and women occur at the highest corporate levels (Thacker, 1995).

Various studies have found similarities in the value placed on career issues by men and women. Gati, Osipow, and Givon (1995) found that men and women place high importance on professional advancement, income, variety, and field of interest. Rowe and Snizek (1995) also found that workers value high income, feelings of accomplishment, and opportunity for advancement. Nonetheless, where they choose to work and how they attribute meaning to different aspects of their jobs can be quite different for men and women (Gati, Osipow, & Givon, 1995; Melamed, 1995).

Work and Other Roles

Gender differences are evident in the impact of multiple roles on men and women. When men add the roles of father or husband, their earnings increase and their employment status increases; however, when women add new roles, their earnings and positions are most likely to remain the same or decrease (Joesch, 1994; Lobel & St. Clair, 1992).

Gender and Success

Melamed (1995) analyzed career success among men and women in England. Successful women tend to work in less competitive and less prosperous environments, and both past education and job experience can affect women's success. In contrast, to be successful, men need the "right" personality profile defined by being outgoing, extroverted, independent, and dominant. Melamed argues that large public-sector organizations tend to employ individuals with these female "success" profiles, whereas male-oriented industries with opportunities for growth and development that require competitive players tend to support the "male" success profile.

In a study of young adults in Israel, Gati, Osipow, and Givon (1995) found that men's career preferences tend to parallel traditional male business and technology orientation, whereas women's preferences tend toward social and humanistic orientations. More profoundly, however, an analysis of responses given by men and women who had been asked to evaluate career aspects of their jobs indicated that men's and women's responses showed different clustering patterns, which indicated that they attribute different meaning to the same aspects of their jobs. The authors underscore the importance of this finding relative to career development theories that assume all career aspects have uniform meaning among workers.

Management Issues

In a biographical study of women in management, Sachs, Chrisler, and Devlin (1992) found that women in management had egalitarian attitudes, had parents supportive of their career choices, had primarily male role models, and were either masculine or androgynous with regard to their gender orientation. Further studies found that whereas women are making significant gains in corporations, they still are not given key assignments involving international relocation, or negotiation roles, or opportunities for managing multiple functions or key business units (Ohlott, Ruderman, & McCauley, 1994).

Tharenou, Latimer, and Conroy (1994) found in a study of Australian managers that on-the-job training was associated with greater advancement for men but not for women. Betz and Fitzgerald's (1987) seminal work on women's career development also indicates that women show fewer gains than men from their educational backgrounds.

In a study of managers in Great Britain, Germany, and the United States, Schein and Mueller (1992) found that successful middle managers had instrumental characteristics more often associated with men than women. In another study, however, Eagly, Karau, and Makhijani (1995) found that male and female leaders and managers may have different behavior styles and yet be equally effective. However, Eagly and colleagues also found that there are gender differences in the positions and organizations in which men and women are most successful. Women are more effective in roles that require interpersonal skills, and men are more effective in positions requiring task ability.

Career Objectives

In contrast to the many differences noted above, there are also similarities in attitudes of men and women toward work-related concerns (see Stoltz-Loike, 1992, 1996). Women and men want to earn money and be productive members of society (Chester & Grossman, 1990; Grossman & Chester, 1990), value power associated with work (Grossman & Stewart, 1990), have similar achievement goals (Chester, 1990; Travis, Phillippi, & Henley, 1991), and expect self-fulfillment from their work (Betz & Fitzgerald, 1987).

Self in Relationship

Traditional models of maturation emphasized the importance of separation and autonomy. More recently, theorists have argued that these models are based on male models of development and may be inappropriate for women because females mature through a different process (Chodorow, 1978; Depuy, 1993; Doherty & Cook, 1993; Gilligan, 1982; Miller, 1976; Tannen, 1990). Female development, these authors suggest, may be more appropriately referred to as relationship-differentiation and emphasizes the articulation of the connection of self to others.

In a review of the literature in Doherty and Cook (1993), the authors argue that a woman's relational nature means that her self-identity is linked to how she is perceived by the significant people in her life. A woman's desire to maintain those connections will influence who she is and who she can become. "It is important to emphasize that this focus on relationship in psychological development says more than that relationships are what women do well; it says that relationships are what women are" (p. 17).

Accepted social values tend to parallel characteristics typically ascribed to men, including autonomy, goal-directed activity, assertiveness, dominance, and competitiveness. The relational perspective suggests that other qualities reflecting connectedness, such as nurturance, caretaking, mentoring, and cooperativeness, must also be valued in adult development.

Women's focus on relationships is evident in all aspects of their lives. Intimate friendships with other women that involve sharing feelings and personal details (Baruch, Barnett, & Rivers, 1983; Josselson, 1987; Tannen, 1990) are important to women, and women's same-sex relationships are emotionally closer than those of men (Worell, 1988). Women expect their concerns for others to be reciprocated and look for social support from other people more often than men do (Worell, 1988). Relationships with children are very important to the life satisfaction of many women (Baruch, Barnett, & Rivers, 1983; Doherty & Cook, 1993) even though many mothers view parenting as having a negative impact on career achievement (Marshall & Jones, 1990; Olson, Frieze, & Detlefson, 1990). Even in their work roles, women can bridge apparent conflicts by redefining their work and interactions with colleagues and subordinates (Grossman & Chester, 1990), thereby reducing what may seem like conflicts between their work roles and relational orientation (Doherty & Cook, 1993).

The fact that women pursue different types of jobs than men do may be related to the greater relational aspects of these jobs (see Forrest & Mikolaitis, 1986) but may also relate to constricted career opportunities because of their generally weaker math and science preparations (Betz & Fitzgerald, 1987; Stoltz-Loike, 1993). Cook (1991) suggests that women may select certain careers and not others because they view the obstacles to career achievement among the latter as overwhelming.

IMPLICATIONS

A broad literature exists that discusses work-family concerns. Men and women hold different expectations of success and experience the conflict between work and family issues differently. Women see success as dependent on career and personal/relational concerns, whereas men see success as related primarily to workplace achievement. Similarly, women spend more time in family roles even when they are employed full-time and experience greater life satisfaction as they increase their family roles.

The profound challenge for both men and women is to find ways to achieve balance among multiple roles. More significantly, it is not how many different roles parents have that contributes to their interrole conflict but rather the *way* that those various roles are balanced and the meaning attributed to *each role*.

Women and men often have different career histories. Women have more discontinuous career paths, and men and women are typically employed in different fields. Even within the same career fields, women and men have different earnings and promotions potential, which is evident almost from the time they begin their employment. It is questionable whether or not the differences are as pronounced among nonparents and among women who have always been employed full-time. Furthermore, women and men may interpret the meaning of particular aspects of work in different ways. Despite these differences, women and men have similar achievement goals, want to be productive and have self-fulfillment from their jobs, and can be equally successful in leadership roles.

The different career histories of men and women have profound implications for their earnings potential, so women typically earn significantly less than men. Erroneous stereotypes regarding women's career commitment may also influence employers' willingness to invest in valuable training and development opportunities for them. More significantly, in terms of this chapter, these results suggest that men and women have profound differences with regard to how they experience work even when they are employed in the same jobs within the same industries.

A final and significant area addressed in this chapter is the way that women define themselves in relation to others. It is only through their significant relations that women arrive at their own self-definition, which is inextricably tied to their relations to significant others. This definition explains why men and women experience such profound differences in their career histories. However, it also raises questions about the implications for women's career development. The world of work is defined in "masculine" terms, such as aggressiveness, individualism, competitiveness, and being results-oriented. Women's greater focus on relational issues contrasts with these characteristics and suggests that women will make a variety of career choices that will remove them from the conflict they experience between the world of work and their concerns with relationships. First, women may self-select for inclusion in traditional male careers. Those women who have more "masculine" gender roles may experience less conflict. Second, women in traditional male careers may spend more time building relations within the work environment with colleagues, subordinates, and clients, to express their relational sides. Third, women may self-select for traditionally female careers. Fourth, women may become entrepreneurs so that they can create a business environment in which they feel more comfortable. Fifth, as more women enter career areas that have primarily employed men, those fields may change and become more accepting of relational components. Sixth, cross-cultural pressures may lead to a change in the traditional American workplace toward putting more emphasis on building relationships and cooperation, which is characteristic of business environments in many other parts of the world.

BALANCE AND SPIRITUALITY

Because the career development literature on spirituality is quite limited, this discussion begins with a working definition of spirituality. *Spirituality is the recognition that we can be influenced by factors that extend beyond the tangible concerns that we have in our daily existence. It reflects the human yearning to touch something significantly greater than ourselves.* Spirituality can be developed from a religious, philosophical, ethical, or moral framework.

Spirituality represents another side of us, and this side grows or shrinks depending on the amount of time we invest in its development. Ideally it should have a *humanizing influence on people*, helping us to understand ourselves better so that we can positively affect other people. Additionally, spirituality can *act as an organizing principle* for the way we function, anchoring us and helping us to place the choices we make and the balance we create within our lives in a meaningful perspective.

Spirituality and Career Choices

As mentioned above, our spirituality can influence the kinds of choices we make. As men and women try to balance multiple role responsibilities, they can begin to ask a number of questions: (1) What are the long-range implications of my choices? (2) How do my choices influence not only my ability to earn money and be with my children but also my ability to develop as a person and as a member of a community and to grow spiritually? (3) How will this choice help me to more fully express other important parts of myself?

At its most profound limit, spirituality allows the full expression of the self, adding another dimension to the way that we normally define ourselves. Ideally it also demands that we retake control of our lives and personal needs.

The gender differences that have been reported throughout this chapter suggest that men and women will experience and express their spirituality differently. Perhaps men will be more accomplished at achieving an intellectual perspective on spirituality but will have difficulty in connecting that sense of self with other people. In contrast, women may be more successful at using spirituality to affect other people yet have more difficulty integrating it intellectually with other aspects of themselves.

My Spiritual Experience

For me, religion is the expression of my spirituality. I was born and raised as an Orthodox Jew, and it is my connection to my religion that has been the organizing principle of my life. Although most people think of the restrictions of organized religion, and they do exist, I consider religion as providing an opportunity for personal expression and the development of my spiritual side.

According to Judaism, the highest level of spiritual expression is the responsibility of every person to be engaged in *tikkun olam,* or bringing positive aspects of development to others. My ability to engage in career, family, and communal and volunteer activities represent my attempt at *tikkun olam.*

I have spent the last twenty years as part of a dual-career couple and the last nineteen years as a parent. I currently have four children. Like everyone else, balancing family and work responsibilities has proved an unbelievable challenge. My involvement in spiritual activities has helped me to find an effective balance.

For example, we observe the Sabbath religiously, which means that I don't engage in work from sundown on Friday until after dark on Saturday. We have always used this as an opportunity to reconnect as a family. That has always meant that no matter how much time has been spent in work-related activities and how few opportunities our family has had to talk to one another, we set aside time to be together on the Sabbath. Because I don't engage in any work, the Sabbath is also a time to visit friends, which helps keep me from getting buried too deeply and permanently under my work. Finally, the Sabbath provides me with time to reconnect with myself by relaxing, reading, or walking.

The idea of stopping all work at least once a week is quite dramatic. I work at a highly demanding job that requires a significant degree of travel and long hours to be successful. It is easy for me to overinvest myself in the importance of the work that I do and to believe that my colleagues and clients cannot function without me. Then the Sabbath or religious holidays come, and I become humbled and also reanchored. I can function without my work, but my organization can also function without me. I remember that I am only an infinitely small part of this vast universe but also that I have important responsibilities beyond my work role.

The various Jewish holidays that occur throughout the year, which we also observe quite strictly, provide me with an ability to balance the intense demands of my life in a way that I think would be impossible otherwise. Religious holidays provide me with an opportunity for self-reflection and allow me to become reenergized by requiring me to rest and stop working. I make the time to question myself, think of where I am going, what my goals are, what I am doing, and how I am developing.

This relates to another aspect of religion that has profound significance for me and involves the need to recognize that the impact of my actions has reverberations beyond myself. I feel myself obligated to be part of community and volunteer activities in another attempt at *tikkun olam,* because I may have knowledge, abilities, or skills that could help others and it is my responsibility to get involved.

Although Judaism advocates self-improvement, there also is a constant emphasis on the importance of balance in people's lives. Maimonides, the great Jewish scholar who lived in the twelfth century, spoke about the "golden path," which he defined as the midpoint between any two extremes of behavior. The goal for people is to constantly look for that middle road. Those individuals who are sensitive to the needs of others should also take time to learn about religious issues, and conversely, scholars must also take time to be concerned with the needs of other people. In Proverbs 1:8, children are admonished to learn about the philosophy of religion from their fathers and the laws and strictures from their mothers, because they need to understand both aspects of religion.

This approach to balance is associated with gender differences. Men and women may exhibit a variety of different behaviors across situational variables. The perspective of Judaism is that successful people can effectively employ both types of behavior, and it is the obligation of the successful religious person to do so. In particular, with regard to family relations, men are admonished to be supportive and to use active listening skills with their wives and children; in other words, to develop and use their expressive sides. Women are expected to have a profound impact on teaching their children about fundamental issues of Jewish law, a reflection of task-orientation.

The great Jewish sage Hillel, who lived approximately two thousand years ago, said, "If I am not for myself, who will be for me? If I am for myself alone, what am I? If not now, when?" This statement parallels both gender difference issues and the need for creating balance within oneself. First, Hillel suggests the importance of individuality. Individuals need to be concerned with themselves and their own needs. Next, however, individuals must be able to see themselves as "I in relationship to others," because we are worthless if all we are concerned with is ourselves. Further, the connection between the two statements suggests that there is an active dynamism, a constant concern with balance between personal needs and the need to relate to other people. Finally, intellectual understanding is not good enough. It must be combined with action toward self-development, helping others, and being a productive member of the community.

There is a story about a famous rabbi named Yochanan who was about to die. The rabbi was a scholar and also a righteous man. When his students came to visit him, he began to cry. His students were quite confused. Here was their revered rabbi, who should have no fear of death; why would he cry? In an attempt to comfort him, his students asked him why he cried. "You are as wise and saintly as Moses and the patriarchs." The rabbi told them, "I know that when I ascend to heaven, God will not ask me why I have not been as good or as wise as Moses. I will be asked why I have not been as good or as wise as Yochanan could have been, why I have not done all that Yochanan could have done, and that is what I fear."

This story represents the challenge of expressing one's own spirituality. The goal is to define ourselves and to take advantage of the unique endowments that we have, to be involved in improving ourselves and the world in which we live.

REFERENCES

Anderson, C. D., & Tomaskovic-Devey, D. (1995). Patriarchal pressures: An exploration of organizational processes that exacerbate and erode gender earnings inequality. *Work and Occupations, 22,* 328–356.

Barker, K. (1993). Changing assumptions and contingent solutions: The costs and benefits of women working full- and part-time. *Sex Roles, 28,* 47–71.

Barnett, R. C., Raudenbush, S. W., Brennan, R. T., Pleck, J. H., & Marshall, N. L. (1995). Changes in job and marital experiences and change in psychological distress: A longitudinal study of dual-earner couples. *Journal of Personality and Social Psychology, 69,* 839–850.

Baruch, G., Barnett, R., & Rivers, C. (1983). *Lifeprints.* New York: Signet.

Beckwith, J. B. (1992). Stereotypes and reality in the division of household labor. *Social Behavior and Personality, 20,* 283–288.

Benin, M. H., & Agostinelli, J. (1988). Husbands' and wives' satisfaction with the division of labor. *Journal of Marriage and the Family, 50,* 349–361.

Berardo, D. H., Shehan, C. L., & Leslie, G. R. (1987). A residue of tradition: Jobs, careers, and spouses' time in housework. *Journal of Marriage and the Family, 49,* 381–390.

Betz, N. E., & Fitzgerald, L. F. (1987). *The career psychology of women.* Boston: Academic Press.

Bird, G. W., & Ford, R. (1985). A source of role strain among dual-career couples. *Home Economics Research Journal, 14,* 187–194.

Blair, S. L., & Johnson, M. P. (1992). Wives' perceptions of the fairness of the division of household labor: The intersection of housework and ideology. *Journal of Marriage and the Family, 54,* 570–581.

Brintnell, E. S., Madill, H. M., Montgomerie, T. C., & Stewin, L. L. (1992). Work and family issues after injury: Do female and male client perspectives differ? *Career Development Quarterly, 41,*145–160.

Bronfenbrenner, U., & Crouter, A. C. (1982). Work and family through time and space. In S. B. Kammerman & S. D. Hayes (Eds.), *Families that work.* Washington, DC: National Academy Press.

Chester, N. L. (1990). Achievement motivation and employment decisions: Por-traits of women with young children. In H. Y. Grossman and N. I. Chester (Eds.), *The experience and meaning of work in women's lives.* Hillsdale, NJ: Erlbaum.

Chester, N. L., & Grossman, H. Y. (1990). Introduction: Learning about women and their work through their own accounts. In H. Y. Grossman and N. I. Chester (Eds.), *The experience and meaning of work in women's lives.* Hillsdale, NJ: Erlbaum.

Chodorow, N. (1978). *The reproduction of mothering.* Berkeley: University of California Press.

Cook, E. P. (1991). Annual review: Practice and research in career counseling and development, 1990. *Career Development Quarterly, 40,* 99–131.

Cotton, S., Antill, J. K., & Cunningham, J. D. (1990). The work attachment of mothers with preschool children. *Psychology of Women Quarterly, 14,* 255–270.

Coverman, S., & Sheley, J. F. (1986). Changes in men's housework and child-care time: 1965–1975. *Journal of Marriage and the Family, 48,* 413–422.

Danser, S. L., & Gilbert, L. A. (1993). Spouses' family-work participation and its relation to wives' occupational level. *Sex Roles, 28,* 127–145.

Depuy, P. (1993). Women in intimate relationships. In E. P. Cook (Ed.), *Women, relationships, and power: Implications for counseling.* Alexandria, VA: American Counseling Association.

Doherty, P. A., & Cook, E. P. No woman is an island: Women and relationships. In E. P. Cook (Ed.), *Women, relationships, and power: Implications for counseling*. Alexandria, VA: American Counseling Association.

Duncan, K. C., Prus, M. J., & Sandy, J. G. (1993). Marital status, children, and women's labor market choices. *The Journal of Socio-Economics, 22,* 277–288.

Eagly, A. H., Karau, S. J., & Makhijani, M. G. (1995). Gender and the effectiveness of leaders: A meta-analysis. *Psychological Bulletin, 117,* 125–145.

Farmer, H. S., Wardrop, J. L., Anderson, M. Z., & Risinger, R. (1995). Women's career choices: Focus on science, math, and technology careers. *Journal of Counseling Psychology, 42,* 155–170.

Felmlee, D. H. (1995). Causes and consequences of women's employment discontinuity, 1967–1973. *Work and Occupations, 22,* 167–187.

Forrest, L. (1994). Career assessment for couples. *Journal of Employment Counseling, 31,*168–187.

Forrest, L., & Mikolaitis, N. (1986). The relational component of identity: An expansion of career development theory. *Career Development Quarterly, 35,* 76–88.

Gassin, E. A., Kelly, K. R., & Feldhusen, J. F. (1993). Sex differences in the career development of gifted youth. *The School Counselor, 41,* 90–95.

Gati, I., Osipow, S. H., & Givon, M. (1995). Gender differences in career decision making: The content and structure of preferences. *Journal of Counseling Psychology, 42,* 204–216.

Gilligan, C. (1982). *In a different voice.* Cambridge, MA: Harvard University Press.

Glass, J., & Fujimoto, T. (1995). Employer characteristics and the provision of family responsive policies. *Work and Occupations, 22,* 380–411.

Greenberger, E., Goldberg, W. A., Crawford, T. J., & Granger, J. (1988). Beliefs about the consequence of maternal employment for children. *Psychology of Women Quarterly, 12,* 35–59.

Grossman, H. Y., & Chester, N. L. (1990). *The experience and meaning of work in women's lives.* Hillsdale, NJ: Erlbaum.

Grossman, H. Y., & Stewart, A. J. (1990). Women's experience of power over others: Case studies of psychotherapists and professors. In H. Y. Grossman and N. I. Chester (Eds.), *The experience and meaning of work in women's lives.* Hillsdale, NJ: Erlbaum.

Guelzow, M. G., Bird, G. W., & Koball, E. H. (1991). An exploratory path analysis of the stress process for dual-career men and women. *Journal of Marriage and the Family, 53,* 151–164.

Hanson, S. L., & Sloane, D. M. (1992). Young children and job satisfaction. *Journal of Marriage and the Family, 54,* 799–811.

Hazard, L. B., & Koslow, D. (1986). Conjoint career counseling: Counseling dual-career couples. In Z. Leibowitz & D. Lea (Eds.), *Adult career development: Concepts, issues, and practices* (pp. 171–186). Alexandria, VA: National Career Development Association.

Hiller, D. V., & Dyehouse, J. (1987). A case for banishing "dual-career" marriages from the research literature. *Journal of Marriage and the Family, 49,* 787–795.

Hiller, D. V., & Philliber, W. W. (1986). Determinants of social class identification for dual-earner couples. *Journal of Marriage and the Family, 48,* 583–587.

Hoffman, L. W., & Nye, F .I. (1974). *Working mothers.* San Francisco: Jossey-Bass.

Hojat, M., Gonnella, J. S., & Xu, G. (1995). Gender comparisons of young physicians' perceptions of their medical education, professional life, and practice: A follow-up study of Jefferson Medical College graduates. *Academic Medicine, 70,* 305–312.

Horst, E. A. (1995). Reexamining gender issues in Erikson's stages of identity and intimacy. *Journal of Counseling & Development, 73,* 271–278.

Hughes, D. L., & Galinsky, E. (1994). Gender, job and family conditions, and the psychological symptoms. *Psychology of Women Quarterly, 18,* 251–270.

Hyde, J. S., Klein, M. H., Essex, M. J., & Clark, R. (1995). Maternity leave and women's mental health. *Psychology of Women Quarterly, 19,* 257–285.

Joesch, J. M. (1994). Children and the timing of women's paid work after childbirth: A further specification of the relationship. *Journal of Marriage and the Family, 56,* 429–440.

Josselson, R. (1987). *Finding herself: Pathways to identity development in women.* San Francisco: Jossey-Bass.

Kirchmeyer, C. (1993). Nonwork-to-work spillover: A more balanced view of the experience and coping of professional women and men. *Sex Roles, 28,* 531–552.

Levine, P. B., & Zimmerman, D. J. (1995). A comparison of the sex-type of occupational aspirations and subsequent achievement. *Work and Occupations, 22,* 73–84.

Light, H. K. (1984). Differences in employed women's anxiety, depression, and hostility levels according to their career and family role commitment. *Psychological Reports, 55,* 290.

Lips, H. M. (1992). Gender- and science-related attitudes as predictors of college students' academic choices. *Journal of Vocational Behavior, 40,* 62–81.

Lobel, S. A. (1991). Allocation of investment in work and family roles: Alternative theories and implications for research. *Academy of Management Review, 15,* 507–521.

Lobel, S. A., & St. Clair, L. (1992). Effects of family responsibilities, gender, and career identity salience on performance outcomes. *Academy of Management Journal, 35,* 1057–1059.

Loerch, K. J., Russell, J. E., & Rush, M. C. (1989). The relationship among family domain variables and work-family conflict for men and women. *Journal of Vocational Behavior, 35,* 288–308.

Loscocco, K. A., & Roschelle, A. R. (1991). Invited contribution: Influences on the quality of work and nonwork life: Two decades in review. *Journal of Vocational Behavior, 39,* 185–225.

Luzzo, D. A. (1994). Ethnic group and social class differences in college students' career development. *Career Development Quarterly, 41,*161–173.

Mackey, W. C. (1995). U.S. fathering behaviors within cross-cultural context: An evaluation by an alternate benchmark. *Journal of Comparative Family Studies, 26,* 443–458.

Marshall, M. R., & Jones, C. H. (1990). Childbearing sequence and the career development of women administrators in higher education. *Journal of College Student Development, 31,* 531–537.

McGowen, K. R., & Hart, L. E. (1992). Exploring the contribution of gender identity to differences in career experiences. *Psychological Reports, 70,* 723–737.

McHale, S. M., & Crouter, A. C. (1992). You can't always get what you want: Incongruence between sex-role attitudes and family work roles and its implications for marriage. *Journal of Marriage and the Family, 54,* 537–547.

Melamed, T. (1995). Career success: The moderating effect of gender. *Journal of Vocational Behavior, 47,* 35–60.

Miller, J. B. (1976). *Toward a new psychology of women.* Boston: Beacon Press.

Morgan, S., Schor, S. M., & Martin, L. R. (1993). Gender differences in career paths in banking. *Career Development Quarterly, 41,* 375–382.

Morgan, K. C., & Hock, E. (1984). A longitudinal study of psychosocial variables affecting the career patterns of women with young children. *Journal of Marriage and the Family, 46,* 383–390.

Nakhaie, M. R. (1995). Housework in Canada: The national picture. *Journal of Comparative Family Studies, 26,* 409–425.

Napholz, L. (1995). Indexes of psychological well-being and role commitment among working women. *Journal of Employment Counseling, 32,* 22–31.

Nettles, K. D. (1995). Home work: An examination of the sexual division of labor in the urban households of the East Indian and African Guyanese. *Journal of Comparative Family Studies, 26,* 427–441.

Ohlott, P. J., Ruderman, M. N., & McCauley, C. D. (1994). Gender differences in managers' developmental job experiences. *Academy of Management Journal, 37,* 46–67.

Olson, J. E., Frieze, I. H., & Detlefson, E.G. (1990). Having it all? Combining work and family in a male and a female profession. *Sex Roles, 23,* 515–533.

Perlow, L. A. (1995). Putting the work back into work/family. Special Issue: Organizational Studies Conference: Best papers. *Group & Organization Management, 20,* 227–239.

Philliber, W. W., & Hiller, D. V. (1978). The implication of wife's occupational attainment for husband's class identification. *The Sociological Quarterly, 19,* 450–458.

Pietromonaco, P. R., Manis, J., & Markus, H. (1987). The relationship of employment to self-perception and well-being in women: A cognitive analysis. *Sex Roles, 17,* 467–477.

Pina, D. L., & Bengsten, V. L. (1993). The division of household labor and wives' happiness: Ideology, employment, and perception of support. *Journal of Marriage and the Family, 55,* 901–912.

Potuchek, J. L. (1992). Employed wives' orientations to breadwinning: A gender theory analysis. *Journal of Marriage and the Family, 54,* 548–558.

Reschly, D. J., & Wilson, M. S. (1995). School psychology practitioners and faculty: 1986 to 1991–92 trends in demographics, roles, satisfaction, and system reform. *School Psychology Review, 24,* 62–80.

Rothausen, T. J. (1994). Job satisfaction and the parent worker: The role of flexibility and rewards. *Journal of Vocational Behavior, 44,* 317–336.

Rowe, R., & Snizek, W. E. (1995). Gender differences in work values: Perpetuating the myth. *Work and Occupations, 22,* 215–229.

Rushing, B., & Schwabe, A. (1995). The health effects of work and family role characteristics: Gender and race comparisons. *Sex Roles, 33,* 59–75.

Sachs, R., Chrisler, J. C., and Devlin, A. S. (1992). Biographic and personal characteristics of women in management. *Journal of Vocational Behavior, 41,* 89–100.

Sandqvist, K. (1995). Verbal boys and mathematical girls: Family background and educational careers. *Scandinavian Journal of Educational Research, 39,* 5–36.

Schein, V. E., & Mueller, R. (1992). Sex role stereotyping and requisite management characteristics: A cross-cultural look. *Journal of Organizational Behavior, 13,* 439–447.

Schneer, J. A., & Reitman, F. (1995). The impact of gender as managerial careers unfold. 290–315.

Sears, H. A., & Galambos, N. L. (1992). Women's work conditions and marital adjustment in two-earner couples: A structured model. *Journal of Marriage and the Family, 54,* 789–797.

Sekaran, U. (1986). *Dual-career families.* San Francisco: Jossey-Bass.

Sekaran, U. (1989). Understanding the dynamics of self-concept of members of dual-career families. *Human Relations, 42,* 97–116.

Seron, C., & Ferris, K. (1995). Negotiating professionalism: The gendered social capital of flexible time. *Work and Occupations, 22,* 22–47.

Silverman, L. K. (1995). Why are there so few eminent women? *Roeper Review, 18,* 5–13.

Spiker-Miller, S., & Kees, N. (1995). Making career development a reality for dual-career couples. *Journal of Employment Counseling, 32,* 32–45.

Stohs, J. H. (1992). Career patterns and family status of women and men artists. *Career Development Quarterly, 40,* 223–233.

Stohs, J. H. (1995). Predictors of conflict over the household division of labor among women employed full-time. *Sex Roles, 33,* 257–275.

Stoltz-Loike, M. (1992). *Dual career couples: New perspectives in counseling.* Alexandria, VA: American Association for Counseling and Development.

Stoltz-Loike, M. (1993). Balancing relationships with careers. In E. P. Cook (Ed.), *Women, relationships, and power: Implications for counseling.* Alexandria, VA: American Counseling Association.

Stoltz-Loike, M. (1996). Annual Review: Practice and research in career development and counseling, 1995. *Career Development Quarterly,* in press.

Tannen, D. T. (1990). *You just don't understand.* New York: Morrow.

Terwillinger, J. S., & Titus, J .C. (1995). Gender differences in attitudes and attitude changes among mathematically talented youth. *Gifted Child Quarterly, 39,* 29–35.

Tesch, B. J., Osborne, J., Simpson, D. E., Murray, S. F., & Spiro, J. (1992). Women physicians in dual-physician relationships compared with those in other dual-career relationships. *Academic Medicine, 67,* 542–544.

Thacker, R. A. (1995). Gender, influence tactics, and job characteristics preferences: New insights into salary determination. *Sex Roles, 32,* 617–638.

Tharenou, P., Latimer, S., & Conroy, D. (1994). How do you make it to the top? An examination of influences on women's and men's managerial advancement. *Academy of Management Journal, 37,* 899–931.

Thompson, L., & Walker, A. J. (1989). Gender in families: Women and men in marriage, work, and parenthood. *Journal of Marriage and the Family, 51,* 845–871.

Tiedje, L. B., Wortman, C. B., Downey, G., Emmons, C., Biernat, M., & Lang, E. (1990). Women with multiple roles: Role-compatibility perceptions, satisfaction, and mental health. *Journal of Marriage and the Family, 52,* 63–72.

Travis, C. B., Phillippi, R. H., & Henley, T. B. (1991). Gender and causal attributions for mastery, personal, and interpersonal events. *Psychology of Women Quarterly, 15,* 233–249.

Voydanoff, P. (1988). Work role characteristic, family structure demands, and work/family conflict. *Journal of Marriage and the Family, 50,* 749–761.

Wilson, M. S., & Reschly, D. J. (1995). Gender and school psychology: Issues, questions, and answers. *School Psychology Review, 24,* 45–61.

Williams, J. C. (1990). Sameness feminism and the work/family conflict. *New York Law School Law Review, 35,* 347–360.

Williams, K. J., & Alliger, G. M. (1994). Role stressors, mood spillover, and perceptions of work-family conflict in employed parents. *Academy of Management Journal, 37,* 837–868.

Worell, J. (1988). Women's satisfaction in close relationships. *Clinical Psychology Review, 8,* 477–498.

Yogev, S., & Brett, J. (1985). Perceptions of the division of housework and child-care and marital satisfaction. *Journal of Marriage and the Family, 47,* 609–618.

Zhang, C., & Farley, J. E. (1995). Gender distribution of household work: A comparison of self-reports by female college faculty in the United States and China. *Journal of Comparative Family Studies, 26,* 195–205.

CHAPTER EIGHT

Vocation as Calling

Affirmative Response or "Wrong Number"

Carole A. Rayburn
Independent Practice, Silver Spring, MD

Iᴛ ɪs ᴏɴᴄᴇ again the beginning of our work week. As we are setting our minds to the tasks at hand, our thoughts may wander to the reasons why we are working, what motivates us to work. We may think of the salary that we are getting, occupying ourselves with meaningful activity that fights boredom, achieving and accomplishing some desired goal, being a player in the power games of the corporate world, establishing self-identity or enhancing our egos, attaining a childhood or parental dream of success, helping others in some significant way, becoming more financially and personally secure, or giving a purposeful meaning to life.

Reflecting upon how we view our work may bring us back to basic questions: What is the meaning of life? Why was I born? What is my purpose for being alive? What is my destiny? How do I relate to other people and to the environment? What should I be doing for the better welfare of others? "Work" has often been seen as "doing," "acting," "fulfilling a task." It is recognized by most people that work is usually not done in isolation from others but rather in relationship to others, servicing them in some needed and meaningful way. Yet we may not initially explore our work or vocation as a calling.

This chapter will explore the meaning of "vocation" and "calling," considering the integration of spirituality and work. In our quest for meaning, we search for answers to our ultimate questions: *who* we are, *who* we are divinely called to be, *what* we are called to do for God and others, and *how* we are divinely called to become ourselves in God. Barriers to affirmatively answering a true call to vocation are identified and discussed. In making connections between spirit and career, we will also examine what indicates a "wrong number" in answering a call to vocation and what facilitates an affirmative response to a call that is the "right number." In our search, our quest for meaning in career and spirituality, we will hopefully follow the path to greater self-understanding, self-acceptance, and a sense of being in divine relation with the universe, the good, the transcendent. We will learn that career can have an essence, a spirituality, a creative or life energy that goes beyond the confines of a 9–5 workday.

WHAT IS "VOCATION"?

Vocation, from the Latin *vocare,* "to call," originally meant "a call." The concept came to mean "a call from God." According to the church in the Middle Ages, everyone had a specific place in life, ordained by God. In this society, individuals unquestioningly accepted the position in life divinely ordained for them, serving God in any task, no matter how menial. Distinct lines were drawn between the clergy and the sacred world, and the laity and the secular world. The laity had a vocation, but one thought to be of a lower status than that of the clergy. With Luther and the Protestant Reformation came affirmation of the "priesthood of all believers," with clergy and laity each having an equally valued calling from God. Serving God faithfully in work, with obedience stressed, was of utmost importance (Kee & Shroyer, 1962). Essential to the concept of all work being of equal value is whether the work makes a positive contribution to all of society. This concept is similar to the one expressed in I. Corinthians 12:1 and Romans 12:6–8, speaking of gifts and of the human body and its parts functioning for the good of the entire body: All people have at least one divinely given gift or service-related talent, and all bodily parts (all work) function together for the good of the entire body (for the benefit of all people).

"Call" is seen as a summoning from God to which all are asked to obey; people are to respond responsibly in achieving a divine purpose. Kee and Shroyer (1962) discuss the times when a call is not clear nor motives unmixed or of the highest kind when individuals first begin their service. However, gradually a clearer call comes from the challenge of the work and the needs of those to be served.

Nemeck and Coombs (1992) see "vocation" as involving three distinguishable callings interrelated in one complex mystery: (1) *who* we are divinely called to be (self-identity), (2) *how* we are divinely to become ourselves in our creator (vocational lifestyle), and (3) *what* we are divinely called to do for our creator and for others (mission or ministry). Of course, answering a call also depends upon a certain degree of readiness to discern the call and to be willing to courageously respond to it. God (or whatever an individual holds to be the superior being or force in life) may see us in a way that we do not see ourselves and may be molding us into the persons who will be ready to affirmatively answer a divine call. The hymn "Have Thine Own Way, Lord" (based on Jeremiah 18:6) expresses this phase of the call preparation well: "Have thine own way, Lord, have thine own way. Thou art the potter, I am the clay. Mold me and make me after thy will while I am waiting, yielded and still" (Pollard, 1902). George Herbert's words and John Wesley's hymn also speak to this preparation period: "Teach me, my God and King, In all things thee to see, And what I do in anything, To do it as for Thee."

A divine call usually involves serving or benefiting others. Farnham, Gill, McLean, and Ward (1991) consider every true call as a call to obey God. *Obedience* comes from the Latin *audire*, "to listen." One who would answer a call must first be open to listening with the ear of discernment, the well-known "third ear." This might involve spiritual discernment, intuition, or simply the willingness and the readiness to listen to the guidance of others who are able spiritually to discern the ways that we are being divinely led. We must listen with the ear, mind, and willing heart to the voice of the divine that is beyond our everyday experiences and being. Then we will be more prepared for the possibilities of greater potential and sense of mission than we thought likely for our lives and our desires.

WHO ARE WE DIVINELY CALLED TO BE?

Dittes (1987), speaking especially of the male perspective, discusses a reworking of the dictum by René Descartes, "I think; therefore I am," to "I work; therefore I am." However, a person is much more than a worker. To change the perception from "I am a worker" to "I am someone who sometimes works" involves giving up an important identity to which one has intensely clung. Dittes connects the pain and emptiness of adolescence— when many feel unconnected with anything, orphaned, lost misfits—with the need to latch onto work as a savior. Then an individual can answer the question, "Who are you?" with "I am a counselor," "I am a lawyer," "I am a fire fighter," and so on. So identified may we be with our occupations, however, that when our work goes wrong and does not bring us the status that it seemed to promise, the child in us cries out, "The emperor has no clothes!" Nonetheless, sans our work outfits and work plans, we are still somebody. Indeed we are children of God (or at the very least, children of the universe).

No particular work, then, is a calling. Rather it is the way in which we live out a faithful response to God in whatever employment or avocation we have. In that all of us are children of God and all have a special calling, what is there to stop us from hearing, obeying, and fulfilling our divine calling? The exclusion and discrimination that are experienced by many females, ethnic minorities, and lesbians and gay males often hamper if not prevent all from answering the call from God.

Van Vuuren (1983) notes that although women are going more into nontraditional vocations, some people believe that women are attempting to "rise above their place in life" or answer a call that is a "wrong number." Such a mistaken belief places women under extreme psychosocial pressure to succeed and to prove themselves. Being under such emotional and societal pressure is not conducive to listening to that inner voice of a calling to vocation. It detracts from a more peaceful mind and thrusts many into an angry, fighting stance of rebellion or even retaliation in an effort to regain or to keep self-esteem and a sense of self-worth. Exclusion and discrimination are antithetical to the idea of becoming a special person for a special mission, which is integral to vocation as calling.

Krueger (1994) also notes that individuals may be prevented from maximum exploration of a calling in a job situation by the racism, sexism, and heterosexism in society. He points out that not even the church is exempt from the painful realities of sexism. The sexism in the religious establishment is also noted by Rayburn (1981, 1985, 1991a, b), Rayburn, Richmond, and Rogers (1986), and Richmond, Rayburn, and Rogers (1988). Female laity, and especially female religious professionals, may be unable to respond affirmatively to a calling that involves a ministerial or rabbinical role or even a role related to the theologically sacred (such as helping in the eucharist service or a bar/bat mitzvah). Even when clergywomen have been ordained and hired by a church or synagogue, some members of their congregation or male clergy may reject or not fully accept them as participants in clerical tasks. For instance, Reform Jewish clergywomen may be able to preside over the service in which an infant female is given a special name (*simit bat,* the service that parallels the *bris* for the infant male), but they are not permitted to sign papers as an official religious witness. An obviously pregnant clergywoman in a mainstream liberal denomination may be seen as a threat to her male senior pastor and to some in the congregation. She is no longer viewed as sexless or nonsensual but as a sexual human being, even though the church itself is pictured as a pregnant woman in the Book of Revelation. For clergywomen, it may be a handicap to be seen as earthy rather than ethereal. The saint/sinner dichotomy imposed upon women by many in society places them in second-class status, potentially limiting their service to others and their accepting their finest calling.

Because theoretically all people have a calling for a special vocation, do all or most people answer their call? Probably not, if they turn away from the vocation in which they have very special talents and skills and from caring for others. Instead they may be motivated *primarily* by financial gain, status, influence, or other forms of self-interest. Although answering a divine calling does not necessarily preclude some of these outcomes—Billy Graham has status, power, and influence worldwide—placing these as the main reasons to seek a certain vocation would seem to rule out the kind of committed life necessary to answer a spiritual calling.

Some individuals may have one talent or spiritual gift, whereas others may have many. People can judge their vocation as having been divinely inspired by the affirmation of others who may praise them for being engaged in that work. They may say, "You are a blessing to me!" or "Thank heaven that I have you to help me in this way!" Enough affirmation given by others in this manner would serve as the biblical test of a spiritual gift: "By their fruits shall you know them." If the vocation is really a calling and the caller is God or the divine, then the respondent is providing a service that is for the good of others and a blessing to all.

Who are we called to be? We are called upon to identify with the divine, the good, to be a servant of God to make a better world for the good of others so they might experience a fuller life lived more abundantly. In this sense, a person may be called to be a police officer, a sanitation worker, an attorney, a secretary, a teacher, a counselor, or anyone else whose vocation is motivated for the good of all people or the majority of people. Obviously if some people are dangerous or harmful to others, they may not benefit those with whom they are working. So it is not the worker but the person motivated to do good—that is who God calls us to be. The one who lives a life dedicated to good, who listens to the divine in little things as well as in big things, is most likely to hear the call and respond affirmatively to it.

WHAT ARE WE CALLED
TO DO FOR GOD AND OTHERS?

As has been mentioned, we are divinely called to serve others in a way that will benefit them. Flow (1993), working as a Christian in a car sales firm, saw a threefold divine call: (1) to salvation, or forgiveness and saving from the results of our sins; (2) to sanctification, or to personal holiness, a transformation or becoming a new self; and (3) to service, to an other-centered life of serving others. Thus there is one call with three dimensions bound together as a unity with no one dimension being the primary focus. The vocation is not the calling; rather, the way persons transcend their work by living faithfully for God in some particular employment: That is their vocation.

Referring to a car dealership, Flow discusses three core values in bearing witness to the divine and giving true meaning to a spiritual calling: (1) extraordinary service to others, (2) development of people, and (3) community building. To achieve these goals, he proposes prayer for spiritual guidance. Truth telling is the foundation for developing trust. Further, Flow holds that many individuals in an unchurched, mobile culture may establish their community life in the workplace: Celebrating birthdays and other special events; sponsoring athletic teams; sending flowers; running company blood banks; cooking Christmas dinners; attending weddings, baby showers, and funerals of co-workers become a large part of their lives.

Heiges (1984) sees vocation not as any occupation but concedes that it may include occupation. He holds that the purpose for which God calls all of us is to bring us out of our isolation, loneliness, and alienation into fellowship or a unique community. To him, a theist's vocation is to glorify God by making the best possible use of the spiritual gifts that have been divinely given. Diehl (1991) observes that people are hungering for the means to connect life experiences to their faith: It is important for individuals to link the world of work to the world of faith.

Some are called to a certain vocation very early in their lives. For example, scripture says that Jeremiah was predestined for his work before birth: Jeremiah 1:5, "Before I formed you in the womb I chose you, before you were born I set you apart; I appointed you as a prophet to the nations." Jeremiah was called in a time of crisis, to give word of hope as well as of judgment on the nation of Judah. He was molded or formed early in life to prepare for this need. Others, such as the prophet Samuel, have been dedicated or strongly influenced by parental guidance or desires to go in certain directions from early childhood. In some of these instances, individuals find that this direction is their "true calling" and continue to answer affirmatively to that choice of vocation.

Yet others think they lack some needed talent, skill, or character for the job to which they have been divinely called. Moses had serious doubts about his abilities (Exodus 4:10–12: "Moses said to the Lord, 'O Lord, I have never been eloquent, neither in the past nor since you have spoken to your servant. I am slow of speech and tongue.' The Lord said to him, 'Who gave man his mouth? . . . I will help you speak and will teach you what to say.'"). Initially such people may lack faith that any necessary skills will be divinely provided when the call is answered affirmatively. Too, we have the example of Jonah, the prophet who tried to flee from his calling to save the people of Nineveh. Caught up with how he would appear to others when God turned away divine wrath and forgave the Ninevites, he desperately wanted to escape this mission to which he was being called. However, even after the experience of being swallowed by a whale, God gave Jonah a second chance to carry out his calling. It was quite difficult for Jonah to comprehend the significance of this calling or even why it was that he had to be sent by God to such a seemingly unworthy people. So it is that a calling can be *salvific* not only to others but to the ones called as well.

Sometimes people are taken from positions of high esteem and brought low. Whether this transition is by divine design or not, God uses this as a learning experience. Consider the case of Moses, who was raised by a pharaoh's daughter in the courts of Egypt, fled from these privileged surroundings after killing an abusive Egyptian, and wandered in the plains of Midian tending flocks of sheep and learning to be more reflective in times of stress. He was being prepared to lead his people out of the wilderness of slavery. Then there was Joseph, the son most favored by his father and looked upon enviously by his many brothers for being so special. Sold into slavery by his brothers, he was spared by divine intervention and saved for a calling that would later ensure the welfare not only of his family but of the Egyptians and Hebrews as well. As long as rebellion or pride turned their focus inward rather than toward God and helping others, they were not ready to answer a call to vocation. This does not mean they were to denigrate or chastise themselves but that they were to look to the larger picture of which they were a part but not the entire subject.

Some individuals have been called to very high positions in which they can do much to save others. Esther was chosen to replace Queen Vashti, whose drunken and perverse husband deposed her. Through guidance from God, the advice of her uncle, and her own strength of character, she was able to save her people from extermination. This was her calling at its finest, to save her people from certain death at the hands of their worst enemy. In doing so, she glorified God and God's divine plan.

At times, we are called to act in ways that are the antithesis of what we had been doing up to that point. Samson, divinely sanctified before birth and called to follow Nazirite ways of keeping himself pure in dietary restraints and other expectations, nonetheless yielded to the temptations of flattery and the trickery of Delilah. In his enslavement at the hands of the Philistines, the blinded Samson heard the voice of the God of his early faith and answered the call to save his people from their enemy. Saul, persecutor of Christ's disciples, was divinely converted and became Paul once he answered the call to lead the new religious movement of Christianity.

In specific instances of a call to vocation, some persons may be called after the first person chosen has turned down the call. For example,

Deborah, a judge (Judges 4–5) in Israel, became the commander-in-chief of the army against the enemies of Israel when Barak refused to answer the call to lead the army in this way. Barak would only lead the forces if Deborah would assume the position at the helm of the army. Saul was chosen by the Israelites to be Israel's king. When Saul turned away from God, God through Samuel appointed David to replace Saul. The results of not continuing to answer this call had disastrous results: Saul put himself, his pride, and his overwhelming ambition before the well-being of his people, and he met with death in his last battle. He had so many opportunities to be true to his calling, but he refused to listen to that still small voice calling him out of the wilderness of self-delusion and into the light of committed caring for the welfare of others. We will not necessarily be punished to this extent by not answering yes to a divine call, but neither will we know the divine joy of a choice not only well made but blessed by spiritual beings. Indeed that is what is held to be the job of the presence of God on Earth, the Holy Spirit or divine guide and teacher who leads us in our everyday lives if we allow this to happen.

Christ, the epitome of one who answered the divine call even to the death, devoted his life to saving all people for all time. Answering a call may be a costly task that results in having as many enemies as friends. However, steadfast dedication to a divine call will bring spiritual blessings and a satisfaction beyond all human understanding.

As mentioned, females have been discriminated against in many ways, often preventing them from answering their spiritual calls. After their husbands had died and when they were left alone to provide for themselves in a time very unfavorable to single women, Naomi wanted to leave her daughters-in-law in their country, Moab. One, Orpah, finally did decide to remain in Moab. Ruth, the other daughter-in-law, chose to return to Bethlehem with Naomi. She answered a divine call to choose her mother-in-law's country and religion. For this answer to God's call, she became an ancestor of Jesus. To have left her home and ventured forth with another woman, as vulnerable as single widowed women were, Ruth had to be listening to the voice of faith calling her out of Moab. People who are called, then, must be willing to step out in faith from a more known and comfortable place to one unknown and potentially uninviting at first.

Mary and Martha were two sisters whom Christ visited. Martha had a calling to be a traditional woman, taking care of the home, preparing food for guests, staying in the kitchen and dining room most of the time. Her sister, Mary, however, often sat at the feet of Jesus, absorbing every word he spoke. Jesus blessed this role, this calling, of Mary. Mary did not need to be a duplicate of her sister but could use, for the benefit of others, the teachings of Jesus. She was one of the witnesses of the newly risen Christ. Not only Mary of Bethany, then, but other women were disciples of Christ, called to spread the word of the divine: Junio, Lydia, Priscilla, and Ana. They braved the prejudices of the times to answer their special call.

Some may be very tempted to answer a spiritual call with "I'm too busy or otherwise committed now. Maybe later . . . Call me again, at some other time." Sometimes this might do, but at other times the timing is such that a person needs to respond within a short time or someone else may be chosen for the job. In emergency situations, there may not be time for hesitation, deliberation, or indefinite postponement. Those called are called to commitment, caring, devotion, dedication, faith, and obedience. People do not need to respond completely without thinking, but they must think with the mind of the spirit of the divine as well as with the human mentality. Self does not need to die, but self cannot kill or dominate over caring for others in the desire to accomplish something of substance.

A call to a specific vocation usually involves a benefit or service to God (or some high supernatural power). Farnham, Gill, McLean, and Ward (1991) point out that merely because a task or endeavor is good or worthy does not indicate that a person is called to do it or should continue doing it. Sometimes doing what is good can be the most serious obstacle to doing something even better. Moses was doing something that appeared good when he was living in the midst of the household of the pharaoh in Egypt. He could have been a blessing to many in that country, particularly those in authority. He was called out of that environment, however, to reach a level of spiritual influence far exceeding anything he could have possibly imagined. The call was not something that he was immediately prepared to accept nor even to psychologically agree to do. But it was the divine call to service of others that needed to be answered affirmatively. The call was an urgent one: It would not be denied, and it would not wait indefinitely.

To many theists, greed is the root of all evil: Greed and pride were the cause of Lucifer, the exemplary angel, falling from grace in heaven and becoming the notorious Satan. Wanting all the glory and all the credit for one's work, being unwilling to share the spotlight or the knowledge to do a job, are ingredients of living a me-only lifestyle—or at least a life filled with self-important and selfish people. The misuse of power is often related to a fear of being exposed as less than others think you are and a fear of being made less when others want to share in your responsibilities.

We are aware that certain jobs are limited in quantity and that competition is fierce for many occupations. Some jobs are defined as having much higher status than others, mainly because they are thought to involve the quality of life and protecting people's ways of living. Who is to say that a hand is less than an eye or that a mouth is greater than a foot? All parts work together for the greatest good of the whole entity. Who is to say that collecting garbage is any less important to the quality of life than operating on a person's nose? Work of almost infinite variety is needed to create life worth living. What is important is not so much the work chosen as the attitude and motivation involved in carrying out the vocation.

Karen and Jean went to the same graduate school in clinical psychology. Both came from hardworking middle-class families with a respect for education. Karen has a younger brother; Jean is an only child. Jean's father died when she was ten years old. Her mother married again when Jean was twelve. The two years that Jean's mother was a single parent and had financial reversals were difficult for Jean. She vowed from that time on to enter a profession that would bring her much status and a comfortable financial gain. Clinical psychology seemed to answer the needs she felt. Karen, however, almost always felt a need to help others. Although she did not shun positions with status, this was not her prime motivation for working in clinical psychology.

Jean considers her job primarily as work that gives her financial independence and some emotional maturity and security, but she does not see her vocation as any kind of calling. Karen, on the other hand, is quite aware of the desire and even the need that she had from childhood to help others. She does see her vocation as a calling from God and believes that she has been led by the Holy Spirit to serve others in her practice of clinical psychology.

The way that the differing motivation translates to Jean's and Karen's therapy and counseling clients is quite dramatic: Because Jean looks at what she does as a job, however dedicated she may be to doing the very best job that she can, she does not think she needs to go beyond the hour-long sessions for which her patients pay. Jean regards her job as done at the end of each group of sessions: The clients, she thinks, get just what they have paid for, no more and no less. Karen, however, will often extend the session beyond the hour if this is psychologically needed. This extension does not depend on the ability of the client to pay for the extra time. Karen prays for her patients and for her own ability to reach them and to help them heal. In fact, she considers the gift of healing a God-given matter. Karen's goal is to help bring out the very best in others, to help them realize their highest potential. She believes this is what God does or wants to do for all of us. Imitating God's goals in this way is one of the greatest blessings of life for Karen.

It is possible to enjoy a job without sensing that it is one's calling. Nonetheless, it is more usual for a vocation to which one is called to be the source of much satisfaction and sense of achievement. Burnout may occur far less often when the vocation is a calling. Temporary setbacks in jobs considered to be spiritually influenced are taken in a more balanced way, less personally, and less blame-avoiding. Doing a job for which one senses a true calling may be more difficult at times because it is sometimes painful and less profitable to be caring and honest with others. The rewards include doing the right thing because it feels right and is the right thing to do and being more at peace with oneself—being better able to sleep at night with a clearer conscience. Answering a divine calling may also lead to identifying with a group of people or with the human family as a whole: The spiritually led person would no more want to do a disservice to others than to have others do a disservice to her or him.

The divinely inspired vocation may benefit some but not others. A police officer may see law enforcement as a duty to protect innocent, law-abiding citizens. In carrying out this duty, the officer may maim or even kill persons who are about to injure or kill others. This may be the officer's true mission in career development. The most difficult part of such a vocation is perhaps defining in each instance who the really innocent people are. So what we are called to do in a divinely inspired vocation is not just doing work that services or benefits others but spiritually being able to discern who these others are. For instance, a criminal may be fiercely loyal to his or her family or to other criminals, but defending criminals against crime fighters or innocent people when they are breaking the law and harming others would most certainly be wrong in the moral as well as the legal sense.

Many professions have a built-in concept or requirement of time set aside to do good for at least a few clients at little or no cost to those persons—the pro bono work of attorneys, psychologists, counselors, physicians, dentists, and others are examples. The clergy certainly have many hours dedicated to this work in their religious setting and in the community at large. Yet such considerations usually serve the relatively few and in themselves do not define a calling to vocation. It is possible at times for even the most wealthy and self-sufficient to need special help from others, the sort of help that even money and influence cannot obtain. So all may be needy sometimes and require the help that only another person listening with the "third ear" and the caring heart can provide.

What makes the difference between a call to nursing versus law enforcement? The legal profession versus psychology or medicine? Each of us, perhaps from quite early in our lives—or certainly by the time we have finished high school or college—has discovered our own special skills and talents. Some of us have good communication skills and get along well with other people. Still others may be less inclined to deal directly with people and are more comfortable with machines, equipment, or technology. Some may prefer to work outdoors, whereas others can only tolerate an indoor job. The individual type of work or the setting is not what determines the calling in vocation. God (or whatever an individual holds to be most sacred and transpersonal) knows where each of us is in terms of career development and life development and uses our skills, talents, experiences, and needs to urge us to serve others in ways that each of us can do best. The answer to what we are called to become is mostly a matter of being willing to form the attitude to help others within our job or work, whether we can do so currently or need additional education or experience. The most important thing in where we find ourselves vocationally is not what we have been trained to do but what we are willing to do with the work for which we have been trained.

HOW ARE WE DIVINELY CALLED TO BECOME OURSELVES IN GOD?

Farnham, Gill, McLean, and Ward (1991), discussing how people discern a call, say, "One sign God might be calling is a certain restlessness, a certain dissatisfaction with things as they are . . . a sense of longing, yearning, or wondering; a feeling of being at a crossroads; a sense that something is happening in one's life, that one is wrestling with an issue or decision; a sense of being in a time of transition; or a series of circumstances that draw one into a specific issue" (p. 11).

It is not necessarily that one is unhappy or dissatisfied with a current job or not functioning well within that work. In fact, the individual may have been working in a particular job so long or doing so well that she or he could do the job almost automatically. There may be a period of boredom in which one asks, "Is there no more to this work? Is this all there is? Can I do something more? What more can I do?" There may be a strong desire for further development in one's career, the need to do more with skills already possessed. People may sense that they are in a period of transition, a time of change. The rationale often given for making such a change is that it allows better use of skills to better serve others.

In Scripture (I Corinthians 7:17), Paul advises, "Let everyone lead the life which the Lord has assigned to him [or her] and in which God has called him [or her]." Paul believed that he was living in the period before the end of the world or of the age, and so he was urging Christians not to change their jobs because the time was short before the Messiah would return. He thought that all should responsibly fulfill the jobs that had been divinely assigned to them. Further, he believed that God calls all of us to a certain life and that we are responsible for finding out what that life is and to live it.

Kee and Shroyer (1962) point out that Paul's society was rather static, whereas current society is very mobile and has many opportunities for vocational choice, especially for people of ability. Most significant in vocational choice are motivation, conduct, direction of the job chosen, and ethical impact of a job upon society. We are called to responsible discipleship, and vocation is part of the tapestry of life. Vocation is our way of obeying a divine call in contributing to the functioning of everyday life. Change, then, may be a function of growth in greater obedience to God and greater awareness of how we can better benefit and serve others.

Ann was a clinical psychologist for all of her professional life. Working at a detention center with inner-city youths, she discovered that she was able to reach her clients through an appeal to their emotions and their spiritual beliefs. The former she dealt with in therapy sessions, and the latter she referred to the chaplains. Often, however, the adolescent came back to her for elucidation of the biblical object lesson or some other theological question. A faithful Protestant who was very active in her church, she was also concerned that sexism so abounded in her church that women going to the minister for vocational advice were directed along very traditional stereotypical lines rather than with respect to their skills and talents. She thought she could better serve these two populations by attending seminary. Quite skilled and well-trained as a psychologist, she nonetheless had a growing sense of being at a crossroads, at a transition point in her career. She was wrestling with the issue of whether she could indeed better serve others by having a degree in ministry. Definitely experiencing a dissatisfaction with things as they were, she wondered whether she could use all of the skills and education she already had in psychology, coupled with a degree in ministry, to reach people in a way that she could not do with psychology alone. Actually Ann had been interested in ministry from a very early age, before she was six years old. Had there not been such a prejudice against women in ministry in her particular religious denomination, she might well have chosen that profession instead of psychology. Admittedly there was some resistance on her part: She knew that ministers were not highly esteemed in all parts of society and certainly did not command high salaries. Further, she thought it might be the height of immodesty to aim for such a sanctified and revered position, especially since men and even some women in society were anything but affirming to women in clergy. After several months of prayer and fasting, she realized she was being called to a vocation in ministry.

Graduating from seminary with top honors, she is still having a struggle as a woman with a ministerial degree in a church with sexist attitudes toward women in ministry. She has been doing as much as she can. This includes responding to the call of a minister whom she knew from her seminary days. He had her come to his church to do therapy with church members who were much in need of psychological intervention. She also counseled him and the rest of the church staff about church problems and staff difficulties. She set up special programs for the church youth, made home visits, preached several sermons, held a church revival with the minister, and actually anointed some of the church members who wanted to rededicate their lives. Members wrote to her for many months after her two weeks in that church, and the minister said that at least two people attending the services at which she preached had joined the church. The minister credited her knowledge of psychology and theology with these events. He affirmed her service by saying she was uniquely able to reach people in a way that he could not by bringing in psychological and theological interpretations and explanations of Scripture for the congregation. He reiterated on several occasions that the people not only liked her but also trusted her. He applauded the rapport she had so quickly established between church members and herself. Indeed this did seem to give evidence of a true call to vocation, despite the hindrance of the sexism in the church hierarchy itself. God can work around such barriers and even soften hard hearts in some instances to see some divine goal accomplished.

This brings up the question of why God chooses to call some people, such as Ann in her difficult denomination, when it would be far easier to just continue calling upon men, who would be met with less resistance. This may be a matter of God wanting all to respond to a spiritual call to vocation and divine thinking not being the same as human thinking. Too, just as each of us has different abilities, each of us can reach different audiences. Not even Billy Sunday, Billy Graham, or Robert Schuller have reached everybody. No artist, musician, therapist, or any other professional has equal appeal for every person who might be influenced by someone in her or his life. In the church setting to which Ann went, several women sensed a call of their own to take more leadership roles in the church and in the community. The male minister had been most encouraging of their doing this. However, what they needed was a strong female role model to give them courage and impetus to step out in leadership in such a conservative religious establishment. Ann was what was needed for that situation, and that was how God used her service. Then, in turn, these women as well as the male minister will lead in ways to better serve and bring out the best in others. So the influence, service, and benefit continue indefinitely.

Van Vuuren (1983) notes that being under pressure to succeed and perhaps to prove oneself may be the most difficult part of accepting freedom of choice or freedom to fulfill oneself and one's goals. The struggle is to know oneself inwardly and to avoid taking on noncharacteristic traits imposed from the outside. Strength to endure this struggle must come from inner peace, which is attained only through prayer or meditation, being one with the divine spirit.

When the divine spirit calls us to vocation, the work may be more humble than we would like or that society would reward. We may be asked to do something that we do not view as our strength, such as Moses being asked to talk to others and not feeling competent to do this. Divine gifts can be given to enable us to function in a vocation to which we are divinely called. God seems more interested in our willingness to respond affirmatively to a call to vocation than whether we have all of the qualifications for the job. Doors can be divinely opened to educational resources and to job sites, but opening hearts and minds to service is much more difficult—even for the divine will. Sometimes the call is not to change a current job but to change the direction, emphasis, or attitude. For instance, a person may be a restaurant owner or a cook in a restaurant and be called to do more for other people in that capacity: helping to feed a group of homeless persons in the community; volunteering time in a soup kitchen to feed the needy; offering cooking classes to new, poor mothers; and taking food for special events to orphanages, hospitals, or nursing homes. Such work, within or in addition to one's vocation, enhances one's performance as a worker and one's membership in the human family of the creator.

BARRIERS TO AFFIRMATIVELY ANSWERING A TRUE CALL TO VOCATION

At times, it is not that we do not hear or understand the call to vocation but that we allow barriers to get in the way of saying yes to the call. Fear of commitment is such a barrier: Making a long-term commitment requires much discipline and dedication to the chosen work. Accompanying this fear may be the fear of following in faith, hesitating to go along spiritual paths because of feeling unworthy of such a vocation/attitude or feeling that the world would not reward such a vocation/attitude very highly. So there might be a fear of disappointing others or being ridiculed or rejected by them. A psychologist, committed to go to seminary for a ministry degree, initially might be misunderstood and ridiculed by colleagues. A retired furrier going back to college to get a doctorate in psychology might similarly be mistreated by former co-workers and friends. In fact, others might see the new vocation as a threat to their own choice of vocation and the former furrier's choice of other work as a rejection of them and their own choice. Then these others might try to invalidate this calling to vocation.

Unbelief or disbelief in divine guidance and spiritual influence in choosing a vocation is another barrier to accepting a call to vocation.

A nonhumanitarian attitude toward others is a similar hindrance: If individuals think they need to account only to themselves, they will not see others as part of the big picture of life. Rather, they must include others in a mutual need to survive difficulties by attacking problems together.

Having the wrong motives in accepting one's vocation is a barrier to affirming a call. Being extremely selfish, greedy, hostile, power obsessed, or conceited; being angry at others for long periods of time; having an unforgiving nature; and not wanting to help others maintains a wall between sensing a call to vocation and answering to it positively. Even in jobs in which direct contact with other people is less common (e.g., engineering, physics, lab technology, animal psychology, zoology, entomology, or chemistry), the primary factor is the responsibility a worker takes in doing the best for others in order to benefit humanity in general. Thus it is the ultimate reason for functioning in a vocation that defines a call to vocation, not the specific job per se.

Prejudices outside the person serve as barriers to accepting a call to vocation. Preconceived ideas as to how individuals should think, look, and act to fulfill certain jobs severely limit who will be able to fill those jobs. However, at times divine intervention intercedes in job decisions. In biblical times, Samuel was led by God to seek out young David to replace Saul as the king of Israel. The Israelites were accustomed to seeing Saul, their first king, as a person of great stature: "As he stood among the people he was a head taller than any of the others. Samuel said to all the people, 'Do you see the man the Lord has chosen? There is no one like him among all the people" (1 Samuel 10:23–24). When Saul failed in his high calling, however, Samuel had to replace him with another leader whom God chose. At first, even Samuel looked upon the outer physical image and thought that one of David's older brothers, Eliab, was God's anointed. "But the Lord said to Samuel, 'Do not consider his appearance or his height, for I have rejected him. The Lord does not look at the things man looks at. Man looks at the outward appearance, but the Lord looks at the heart'" (1 Samuel 16:7). After seven sons of Jesse were brought before Samuel and rejected by God as the new king, the youngest son, David, who was "ruddy, with a fine appearance and handsome features" (16:8–12) was accepted as God's chosen and anointed for the Lord's work.

Prejudices against women and ethnic minorities have interfered with their positively responding to a call to vocation. Discrimination in hiring and advancement in a job has set limits on what some people can do within a vocation. Yet the divine element in all calls to vocation can inspire all wherever they are in their employment and enable them to reach other kinds of potentials.

Sorrow can threaten both to close doors and conversely to open doors to being called for vocation. During times when individuals are experiencing deep losses, such as after the death of a loved one, they may be at their most vulnerable and reachable by spiritual influences. Deep sorrow may lead to terrible anger toward the divine and a turning away from God and any serious listening for a call to vocation. Bitterness and resentment at loss may lead the grieving individual to care very little or not at all about helping others. A healthier response, after mourning or sorrowing is completed, is to reach out to God and answer the call with an affirmative response. This will result in the individual's fulfilling a special vocation. Through sorrow and being brought out of sorrow through faith in the divine healer, we are made more sensitive and more concerned for the sorrow and need for healing of other people. We are rendered more ready to accept a call to vocation.

WHAT INDICATES A "WRONG NUMBER"?

In discerning spiritual gifts, we are told that "by their fruits shall you know them." That is, holy and blessed results are a sign of consecrated workers fulfilling God's plan. If a vocation does not "bear fruit" or have a good and positive outcome (in some ultimate sense), there is some question as to whether it was a legitimate call or response to the call.

In the biblical account of King Saul, we have the tragic story of someone who was called for a very high position and mission, who accepted the call, but who fell from it and was finally rejected by God and replaced with David. When Samuel conveyed to Saul that he was chosen by God to fulfill a very high calling, Saul answered, "But am I not a Benjaminite, from the smallest tribe of Israel, and is not my clan the least of all the clans of the tribe of Benjamin? Why do you say such a thing to me?" (1 Samuel 9:21). Initially Saul thought to reject God's call and to answer with a response that it was the "wrong number." However, as Saul turned to leave Samuel, "God changed Saul's heart, and all these signs were fulfilled that day" (1 Samuel 10:9). Saul went his own way eventually and disobeyed the Lord, and Samuel said, "Although you were once small in your own eyes, did you not become the head of the tribes of Israel? . . . Why did you not obey the Lord?" (1 Samuel 15:17, 19). Saul could only proffer that he had disobeyed because "I was afraid of the people and so I gave in to them" (1 Samuel 15:24). Saul was rejected by God and removed from his vocation as king. The call, when it first went out from God, was the "right number." Saul's affirmative response to the calling to vocation was blessed and, if he had continued to be obedient in his mission, he would have known much contentment in a job well done. He would have been able to declare, as did the apostle Paul, "I consider my life worth nothing to me, if only I may finish the race and complete the task the Lord Jesus has given me. . . . In everything I did, I showed you that by this kind of hard work we must help the weak" (Acts 20:24, 35), and "I have fought the good fight; I have finished the race; I have kept the faith. Now there is in store for me the crown of righteousness, which the Lord, the righteous Judge, will award to me." (2 Timothy 4:7–8).

CONCLUSION

Whatever one's spiritual or humanitarian frame of reference, a call to vocation involves responding to the divine, spiritual, supernatural power or to humanistic beliefs outside oneself to serve, benefit, or save other people. An individual's attitude, the change of heart from a less to a more caring stance, is all-important, not so much the particular job in and of itself.

What most facilitates the positive response to a divine call to vocation is dependence on the spirit outside oneself. Individuals cannot of their own selves do anything, but all good things come from the Lord—or whatever the ultimate good is, as in the creation of all life, from the standpoint of nontheists. People are social beings, and all good is thus ultimately seen in relating positively with others in some mutually beneficial way. Answering a divine call to vocation with a resounding *yes* puts into action the blessed work of serving others. Such an enterprise is symbolic of the vocational partnership of the human and the divine.

REFERENCES

Diehl, W. E. (1991). *The Monday connection: A spirituality of competence, affirmation, and support in the workplace.* San Francisco: Harper San Francisco.

Dittes, J. E. (1987). *When work goes sour: A male perspective.* Philadelphia: Westminster Press.

Farnham, S. G., Gill, J. P., McLean, R. T., & Ward, S. M. (1991). *Listening hearts: Discerning call in community.* Harrisburg, PA: Morehouse.

Flow, D. (1993). A business owner's mission: Working as a Christian in a car sales firm. In R. J. Banks (Ed.), *Faith goes to work: Reflections from the marketplace.* New York: Alban Institute.

Heiges, D. R. (1984). *The Christian's calling.* Philadelphia: Fortress Press.

Kee, H. C., & Shroyer, M. J. (1962). *The Bible and God's call.* Teaneck, NJ: The Methodist Church Interboard Committee on Christian Vocations.

Krueger, D. A. (1994). *Keeping faith at work: The Christian in the workplace.* Nashville: Abingdon Press.

Nemeck, F. K., & Coombs, M. T. (1992). *Called by God: A theology of vocation and lifelong commitment.* Collegeville, MN: Liturgical Press.

Pollard, A. A. (1902, lyrics), with Stebbins, G. C. (1907, music). Have thine own way, Lord. In *United Methodist Hymnal* (1989). Nashville, TN: United Methodist Publishing.

Rayburn, C. A. (1981). Some reflections of a female seminarian: Woman, whither goest thou? *Journal of Pastoral Counseling, 16*(2), 61–65.

Rayburn, C. A. (1985). Promoting equality for women seminarians. *Counseling and Values, 29*(2), 164–169.

Rayburn, C. A. (1991a). Clergywomen, clergymen, and their spouses: Stress in married clergy [Special monograph]. *Psychotherapy in Private Practice, 8*(4), 131–140.

CHAPTER NINE

Spirituality, Intentionality, and Career Success

The Quest for Meaning

Deborah P. Bloch
University of San Francisco

THE NEW YORK TIMES runs a week-long series of articles on the effects of corporate downsizing on businesses, on the communities in which they operate or operated, and on individuals who work or worked for them (Uchitelle & Kleinfeld, 1996; Kleinfeld, 1996; Bragg, 1996; Rimer, 1996; Johnson, 1996; Kolbert & Clymer, 1996; Sanger & Lohr, 1996). Two months later, the paper runs a column entitled "Doublespeak." It gives forty-eight euphemisms for getting fired, from "asked to resign" to "workforce imbalance correction" (Zane, 1996). Numerous books describe the changes in the workplace wrought by new technologies, globalization, and the value of the bottom line. Each book provides its own solutions (for example, Bridges, 1994; Rifkin, 1995; Handy, 1989). The only certainty appears to be uncertainty. In this turbulent sea of change, are there constants of individual action that can be drawn upon to provide anchors of meaningfulness?

In the ancient age of hippiedom—the 1960s and '70s—a frequently heard mantra was "Go with the flow." More recently, a retiring U.S. senator, speaking of the uncertainty of his plans, said, "I feel like I'm a work in progress" (Sciolino, 1996). One can imagine hearing these phrases said with a sigh of resignation connoting self-surrender, a surrender to forces greater than oneself, a passive nonresistance. On the other hand, the tone imagined can hold a hint of bitterness, connoting anger at a perceived theft by others of one's internal locus of control, carrying with it a passive aggression. However, a third possibility is hearing the same phrase, "Go with the flow," with a tone of delight, a tone that suggests full participation in the changing world and, with that participation, the conscious effort to find meaning in the river of life in which I find *myself*.

This chapter examines how one can participate in the full flow of life through the development of practices that draw upon nonlinear and intuitive abilities in addition to the rational approaches ordinarily depended upon. Spiritual practices both current and ancient are discussed as are recent findings in science, particularly subatomic physics or quantum mechanics. These practices are directly related in this chapter to how each individual may find the unique qualities of personal meaningfulness and further how individuals may influence their career paths through resonance with the world around them. The chapter is organized into four sections: (1) How is "meaning in work" defined? (2) How can individuals find that meaning for themselves in the work they are doing? (3) How can individuals actually influence the external world to find jobs or work settings that are more meaningful to them? (4) How can professionals help others in their quest? To answer these questions, I have drawn material from diverse sources—poetry, philosophy, quantum mechanics, and career development theory—to develop and present the approaches to meaningfulness in which I have come to believe.

WHAT IS MEANING?

Meaningfulness in work is derived from a sense of harmony—internal harmony, harmony in relationship to others, and harmony in relationship to the things with which one works. In the poem "Two Tramps in Mud-Time," Robert Frost (1949, pp. 357–359) describes the arrival of two strangers who come to his farm and offer to split wood. Although the narrator of the poem loves the task himself, particularly on the day in early spring when the tramps appear, he recognizes that he is playing at something that is the work of others for pay. He hires the strangers because of their need, but not without some reluctance, and it is in that reluctance that he recognizes one of the needs for harmony in life. "My object in life is to unite/ My avocation and my vocation/ As my two eyes make one in sight." Just as the convergence of sight through the right and left eyes produces depth of vision, so answering the call to a kind of work produces depth of meaning.

The harmony that comes from recognition of a vocation or calling is explored in this book in Huntley's chapter, in which he provides a theological framework to answer the question, "What is meaning?" He identifies four approaches: work as a necessity, work as a good in itself, work as a calling, and work as co-creation. Rayburn's chapter expands on the theme of vocation.

However, harmony is not limited to the sense of having answered a call. Although another poet, Donald Hall (1993), describes a sense of being called to his work, of a poem "beckoning joyously," he also expresses a oneness with the work itself. His description of "absorbedness" filling him from "footsole to skulltop" (p. 41) is offered in the introduction to this book as a possible source of meaningfulness. This sense of "absorbedness" is akin to Mihaly Csikszentmihalyi's (1990) characterization of "flow": "*Flow* is the way people describe their state of mind when consciousness is harmoniously ordered and they want to pursue whatever they are doing for its own sake" (p. 6).

Using both case studies and historic literature, Csikszentmihalyi (1990) explores and rejects the notion that flow is limited only to some higher order of jobs or to Western experience. He compares flow to *yu*, described by the Taoist scholar Chuang Tzu, and concludes, "If my interpretation is true, in the flow experience (or *Yu*) East and West meet: In both cultures ecstasy arises from the same sources. Lord Wen-hui's cook [a story told in Chuang Tzu's writings and retold by Csikszentmihalyi] is an excellent example of how one can find flow in the most unlikely places, in the most humble jobs of daily life. And it is also remarkable that over twenty-three centuries ago the dynamics of this experience were already so well known" (p. 151).

A person cannot feel simultaneously at one with the world and stuck in a meaningless job. In *Zen and the Art of Motorcycle Maintenance*, Robert M. Pirsig (1984) echoes Jung's concept of "being stuck" and suggests the following antidote:

> If you want to build a factory, or fix a motorcycle, or set a nation right without getting stuck, then classical, structured, dualistic subject-object knowledge, although necessary, isn't enough. You have to have some feeling for the quality of the work. You have to have a sense of what's good. That is what carries you forward. (p. 284)[1]

Pirsig's description of a mechanic at work presents the ideal absence of the duality to which he refers. Further, although written earlier, it seems a perfectly concrete example of Csikszentmihalyi's "harmoniously ordered" consciousness:

> One says of [the involved mechanic] that he is "interested" in what he's doing, that he's "involved" in his work. What produces this involvement is, at the cutting edge of consciousness, an absence of any sense of separateness of subject and object. "Being with it," "being a natural," "taking hold"—there are a lot of idiomatic expressions for what I mean by this absence of subject-object duality, because what I mean is so well understood as folklore, common sense, the everyday understanding of the shop. (p. 296)[2]

The possibility of "flow," of "being with it," then, is not limited to any particular job. It cuts across all occupations regardless of their associated socioeconomic status. It cuts across all fields, all occupations, all industries. It has to do with how the individual feels about his or her work.

Two aspects of harmony have been touched upon. The first is the internal harmony people experience when doing the work they feel called to do, when they have united what they really enjoy with what they do for pay. A second source of harmony comes from absorption in the work one is doing. When people feel a sense of identification with the work itself, a loss of separation between the work they are doing and themselves, they produce work of a high quality and feel a sense of oneness with that work. Of course, a feeling of having been called to the work and a sense of oneness with the work are not necessarily unrelated. In fact, the more kinds of harmony one can feel, the more meaningful one believes his or her work to be.

There is a third source of harmony as yet unexplored, and that is the unity that people can experience through their work with other people. Although a great deal is being written on teamwork and participatory governance, in general little has been said about the importance of authentic relationships at work. Yet chapter after chapter in this book incorporates the unity of self and other as a key ingredient in meaningfulness. Seeking harmony with others is the opposite of finding people to meet one's needs. "When we use work or people as a means to an end, then obviously we have no relationship, no communion either with the work or with people, and then we are incapable of love. Love is not a means to an end; it is its own eternity" (Krishnamurti, 1956/1992a, p. 16). Meaningfulness, then, comes from a sense of harmony with others, with those with whom one works, with those who are served by the work, with the community of the workplace, the community of a neighborhood, the community of a profession, craft, or trade, or the community of those called to do similar work.

Harmony, unity, the embracing of duality until it is oneness, are keys to a meaningful life. It is difficult to abandon Cartesian notions of duality—self versus other, person versus thing, body versus mind, work versus pleasure. Yet that is what must happen for meaningfulness to be present. For duality, substitute complementarity (also discussed in David Tiedeman's chapter). Complementarity essentially is the holistic view of what had previously been seen as opposites. In a worldview embracing complementarity, there is no separation of self and other. When something happens to you, it affects me. Although the scientific bases of this belief are only now being discovered, in the Renaissance, John Donne wrote, "No man is an island, entire of itself;/....And therefore, never send to know for whom the bell tolls;/ It tolls for thee." Each aspect of the complementary pair or group only exists meaningfully in the context of the other. "Shape clay into a vessel;/ It is the space within that makes it useful" (Lao Tsu, 1989, p. 13). Meaning is the experience of the harmonious connection to whatever you are doing and to whomever you are working with. There may also be a sense that you have been called to the work and that you are helping to create the universe itself. And through all of this may be the pervasive feeling that what you are doing is good in a general sense, of a high quality, and ethically right.

HOW CAN INDIVIDUALS
FIND MEANING FOR THEMSELVES?

The essential tasks of career development are centered on "self, search, and synthesis" (Bloch, 1989); that is, on identifying the needs, interests, values, and other critical variables of the individual; on understanding the nature of work, occupations, and industries; and on bringing these together. Meaningfulness resides in the act of synthesis. So it may be interesting to see how the synthesis has been approached in classical career development theory. Classical career development theory is usually portrayed as beginning with the work of Parsons (1909) and the synthesis of "true reasoning." As the field developed, theories became more psychodynamic, retaining a relationship both to Parsons' practices and to Lewin's (1935) postulate that behavior is a function of the person and the environment.

Holland's work (1992) has centered on the examination of personality types, the identification of the work environments that foster the behaviors associated with the types, and the attempts by the individual to find congruence between the two. The self, in this theory, can be described in terms of the now familiar hexagon of realistic, investigative, artistic, social, enterprising, and conventional dimensions. The search is in the identification of behaviors associated with successful implementation of the various occupations. This has resulted in the Holland instrument, the *Self-Directed Search,* and its manual of coded occupations. It is the attempt to find congruence that comes closest, in Holland's theory, to the idea of synthesis.

Super (1994) describes his own work as straddling person-environment and life-span development approaches. In both aspects of his work, self-concept plays an important role. In the life-span development approaches, Super (1990) develops the concept of stages of career development, with accompanying developmental tasks and transitions, self-concept and values. To marry my terms and Super's, the individual's synthesis would be described as career maturity.

The social learning theory of career development (Krumboltz, Mitchell, & Jones, 1976; Krumboltz & Mitchell, 1990) concentrates on the generalizations individuals make about their world as a result of their own biological makeup, their direct experiences, the results (or reinforcements) of these experiences, and the vicarious experiences they gain through observation. The generalizations then are the synthesizing mental events.

A fuller discussion of current theories, the relationships among them, and the relationship of theory to practice can be found in Savickas and Walsh (1996), *Handbook of Career Counseling Theory and Practice.* Although the theories presented are valuable in explaining various aspects of the underlying process of career choice, job satisfaction, job retention, and work motivation, I do not believe these theories provide understanding of what meaningfulness is to the individual. Practice follows theory in what Jung might have called the use of "rational methods" (1931/1933, p. 61). Current practice in career counseling relies heavily on the identification of interests, abilities (sometimes called transferable skills), and occasionally values. Instruments including interest inventories, aptitude tests, computer-based questionnaires, and card sorts are utilized to help the individual develop the list of supposedly unique characteristics. The responses to the questionnaires lead to the search of databases of information about occupations. These may include print, visual, or computer-based material or even visits to actual work sites. Talking therapy, or counseling, itself most often centers on identifying and overcoming the barriers that may keep the individual from achieving synthesis, which is seen as making a decision and acting upon it.

The synthesis of decision making and action is qualitatively different from the synthesis of meaning-making. Although career counseling, as described earlier, is undoubtedly valuable, it is insufficient in helping the individual find meaning in life, work, or lifework. Meaning comes from knowledge, and knowledge comes from the connections that are made by the individual between information and an already existing mental framework or model. When knowledge is gained, it either adds to the framework or changes its shape to incorporate that which is new. The work of three philosophers can be drawn upon to elucidate this definition of knowledge. In *Personal Knowledge,* Polanyi (1962) develops a schema of how people turn information to knowledge. The model states that knowledge consists of the recognition and reordering of patterns of information. Polanyi draws an analogy between acquiring knowledge and listening to music: "[T]he particulars of a pattern or a tune must be apprehended jointly, for if you observe the particulars separately they form no pattern or tune" (pp. 56–57). Three concepts proposed by Polanyi are keys to understanding how people acquire and use knowledge. The first is that people are always ready for knowledge. He writes, "There is a purposive tension from which no fully awake animal is free. It consists in a readiness to perceive and to act: to make sense of its own situation both intellectually and practically" (p. 120). The second is that to acquire knowledge one must want to do so because of the belief that this knowledge or information is of use. "We can assimilate an object as a tool if we believe it to be actively useful for our purposes. The same holds true for the relation of meaning to what is meant and the relation of the parts to the whole. The act of personal knowing can sustain these relations only because the acting person believes they are apposite: that he has not made them but discovered them" (p. 63).[3] The importance of seeing relationships, of incorporating new information into relationships, and of using new information to change one's understanding of the relationship itself has also been examined by Bateson (1979), who writes about "the pattern which connects" (p. 8). Bronowski (1978) describes the act of imagination as the opening of a system so that new connections are shown: "Every act of imagination is the discovery of likenesses between two things which were thought unlike" (p. 109). Bateson's connecting patterns may be compared to Polanyi's idea of frameworks. Bronowski's description of imagination can be seen as Polanyi's description of the assimilation of information so it can become knowledge. Therefore it can be said that the creation of knowledge from information becomes an act of imagination for each individual.[4]

It is clear from this discussion that the acquisition of knowledge is highly idiosyncratic. It is a personal, individual, solitary act. "I have shown that into every act of knowing there enters a passionate contribution of the person knowing what is being known, and that this coefficient is no mere imperfection but a vital component of his knowledge" (Polanyi, 1962, p. viii). The personal nature of knowing is nowhere more necessary than in knowing what is meaningful. I can generalize about the relationship of harmony to meaningfulness, but I cannot generalize about the particular harmony that is meaningful to any one person or any group of individual persons. Each individual must carry out this process as a solo performer.

Because of the idiosyncratic nature of knowing, especially of knowing meaningfulness, instruments that purport to help in self-description will not assist the individual in finding meaning in work. No matter how sophisticated, instruments that produce lists, even those that combine the findings of several lists, cannot provide knowledge for two reasons: First, the lists are never truly individualized. By definition, there must be a limited set of possible patterns resulting from the responses of the individual. Although the set of patterns that emerges may be large, it cannot be infinite. The development of patterns that can be replicated is the strength of standardized instruments, but it is their limitation as well when it comes to the discovery of individual meaning. Second, the instruments themselves do nothing to assist the individual in synthesizing the information provided. At best, instruments can only be a step in gathering information. They cannot provide, produce, or provoke meaning.

The way to meaning is not passive. It is through actions that put the seeker in touch with aspects of the self that cannot be recognized through other means. At the 1996 California Career Conference, Richard Bolles, in his keynote address, described how a friend found meaning. Each evening, Bolles explained, his friend sits in front of a blank wall—an imagined movie screen—for an hour. In his mind, he plays the events of his day as if they were a movie on the screen. From that movie of his day comes the meaning of his actions and thoughts during that day. Bolles's friend has practiced stillness.

Stillness has been called meditation or mindfulness. It sounds simple, but it is difficult to practice. Stillness requires the discipline of doing nothing in a life that is otherwise filled with action. Once more, the complementarity principle is at work. Here is how the Canadian writer Robertson Davies (1977) describes it in a marvelous essay, "What Every Girl Should Know":

> Whoever you are, your energies and your opportunities are unlimited. Of course you want to try several alternatives in order to find out what suits you, but I hope that ten years from today you will agree with me that the good life is lived not widely, but deeply. It is not doing things, but understanding what you do that brings real excitement and lasting pleasure.

Davies then he goes on to ask how you are to avoid the fate of living without meaning, of not understanding what you do. And he answers:

> I can tell you, but it is not a magic secret which will transform your life. It is very, very difficult. What you must do is to spend twenty-three hours of every day of your life doing whatever falls in your way, whether it be duty or pleasure or necessary for your health and physical well-being. But—and this is the difficult thing—you must set aside one hour of your life every day for yourself, in which you attempt to understand what you are doing.

Davies further discusses this set-aside hour a day in terms of prayer. He draws distinctions among three purposes of prayer: petition, "which is for yourself"; intercession, "which is for others"; and contemplation, "which is listening to what is said to *you*." His final advice is to "stick to petition in the form of self-examination, and to contemplation, which is waiting for suggestions from the deepest part of you" (pp. 50–52).[5]

This practice in many traditions is often called meditation. Stillness as a practice often seems strange to Western minds. There's a two-line joke that seems to tell it all. The Western teacher urges the students, Don't just sit there, do something. The Eastern teacher urges, Don't just do something, sit there. But how does one just sit there? I will provide an exercise at the end of this section, but this description from Krishnamurti (1974/1992c) is the most beautiful, brief set of directions I have seen:

> Sit very quietly and be still not only physically, not only in your body, but also in your mind. Be very still and then in that stillness, attend. Attend to the sounds outside this building, the cock crowing, the birds, somebody coughing,

somebody leaving. Listen first to the things outside you, then listen to what is going on in your mind. And you will then see, if you listen very very attentively, in that silence, that the outside sound and the inside sound are the same. (p. 86)[6]

When stillness is practiced, harmonious order is recognized. Harmony and meaningfulness are one. Krishnamurti described the harmony of the seekers with the world outside themselves—"the outside sound and the inside sound are the same." Those who practice stillness or meditation for medical reasons find the same experience. Many Western-trained physicians have prescribed meditation as a way of healing oneself. Recently Dean Ornish's program for healing heart patients was accepted for compensation by a major insurer. Meditation is one of the key elements of the program. The now well-known practices of the relaxation response originated at the Harvard Medical School. The popular doctor-author Deepak Chopra (1989), who is trained in both Western medicine and *ayurvedic* practice, describes the benefits of transcendental meditation through his work. But what is pertinent to this chapter is the harmonious, self-informing product of stillness. Chopra draws the crucial distinction between the importance of information and its hold on each person's mind, often to the detriment of knowledge. He tells this story as an example:

> A verse from an ancient Indian Upanishad describes this beautifully: "A man is like two doves sitting in a cherry tree. One bird is eating of the fruit while the other silently looks on." The bird who is the silent witness stands for that deep silence in everyone, which appears to be nothing at all when in reality it is the origin of intelligence. (p. 149)

Pelletier (1977), a Western-trained psychologist, advises meditation to reduce stress-related disease. However, he also describes these effects:

> After long practice of a meditative discipline, through which the practitioner has achieved total stilling of the mind and total loss of self as a separate entity, during the meditation, he or she becomes open to a whole new order of reality. At this point, he is pervaded with overwhelming and joyous knowledge that all of existence is a unity that he is at one with and one and the same as all else about him. There is no subject or object, no I or Thou, no Yin or Yang. With this powerful feeling comes a dissolution of all fear, including fear of death, and an inundation of warmth, joy, harmony, and absolute knowledge that there is an order to the universe. (pp. 225–226)[7]

Thus one experiences the absence of subject-object duality identified by Pirsig, the sense of harmonious order described by Csikszentmihalyi. With this sense of order comes a sense of meaningfulness in one's life or a sense of where meaning can come from. Spirituality is a way of knowing that comes from quiet self-examination without thinking. That is the paradox: It is a conscious nonthinking.

It must be stressed that the practice of stillness, or meditation, is not to be seen as a means of avoiding life. The purpose of meditation is not to separate oneself from active life, only to separate oneself for that time. Mindfulness is a way of finding the authentic self in action. It is a way of finding how work has meaning and of bringing meaning to the work. Ueland (1987), writing about her work—and making suggestions to others about the art of theirs—writes, "And it is Tolstoi who showed me the importance of being idle—because thoughts come so slowly. For what we write today slipped into our souls some *other* day when we were alone and doing nothing" (p. 36). Conditioned responses often dominate both lives and work. People see no way of doing things differently, of doing different things, of feeling differently about what they have done, are doing, will do. Caught in spirals of stimulus and response, the lack of meaning is not even felt. "Freedom from conditioning comes with the freedom from thinking. When the mind is utterly still, only then is there freedom for the real to be" (Krishnamurti, 1958/1992b, p. 90). In three questions, Rabbi Hillel distilled both the need for harmony—the connection of self and other—and the need for active expression of the harmony, the "nowness" of action. He asked, "If I am not for myself, who will be for me? If I am for myself alone, what am I? If not now, when?"

▼ Exercise 1   *Beginning Mindfulness: A Sample Practice*

Here then is a practice to begin mindfulness. Before you begin, set a timer for ten minutes. Sit in a comfortable chair with a firm back or on the floor with your back straight and your legs crossed comfortably. Place your hands on your thighs, palms up and slightly open. Straighten yourself as if you were about to pay attention. Now let your shoulders drop naturally. Breathe slowly, in through your nose and out through your mouth. You may make a sound with your breath as you exhale. That's fine. Just breathe in and out deeply and evenly for a few moments. Let your breath return to normal.

Begin to feel the power of the Earth wherever your body is in contact with the floor or chair. Maintain your contact with the abundant power of the physical, material world. Let the energy of the brown and red earth, its dryness, its moist fertility enter your body. Keep the Earth's energy within you. At the same time, become aware of the top of your head. Imagine you can feel the electricity of all the spirit in the cosmos. As you draw in one breath, draw in the abundance of the Earth. As you draw in the next, draw in the light of the cosmos. Picture this as you breathe in and out. Continue to breathe naturally. Simply follow the path of each breath in and out. If you hear sounds or smell anything, note it and let it pass away as you continue to return to a focus on your breathing. Thoughts will cross your mind. Do not become fretful about them. Notice them as thoughts, just as you noticed the external sounds, and allow them to pass across your mind. Any time you lose your concentration in the exercise, just return to your breathing. When the timer rings, slowly open your eyes. As you become more comfortable with this mindfulness exercise, you may want to expand the time gradually.[8] ▲

Mindfulness can be practiced in all arenas and activities of life. *Wherever You Go, There You Are: Mindfulness Meditation in Everyday Life* (Kabat-Zinn, 1994) is an excellent guide. Other techniques that still the daily chatter of active minds may also facilitate the sense of harmony and the growth of spirit. Listening to music, dancing, practicing an art, reading poetry, or letting oneself "get lost" in a picture can also contribute to the sense of oneness that gives meaning to life. The story-telling techniques that Savickas describes in Chapter 1 in this book are counseling tools that can also help the individual toward the experience of harmony.

Finding meaning requires spiritual work. Personal knowledge does not come through casual or unsustained practice. Frost (1949, p. 276) portrays the person who peers into the well and always sees only his own reflection until, just once, a pebble disturbs this vision of self and reveals something more, "For Once, Then, Something." Meditation can produce those moments of pebble disturbance in the routine of daily lives. Again, from the Tao, "Knowing others is wisdom;/ Knowing the self is enlightenment./ Mastering others requires force;/ Mastering the self needs strength" (Lao Tsu, 1989, p. 35).

HOW CAN INDIVIDUALS
FIND WORK THAT HAS MEANING?

In the search for meaningfulness in work, one may discover the need to change how one performs on the job, to change jobs, or even to shift occupations. Traditional assistance with career development, changes in life stages, and external economic circumstances may also suggest or dictate the need for change. In bringing about change, the practice of intentionality is a spiritual approach that can enhance the possibilities for success. The practice of intentionality is the use of the mind to influence events in the world outside oneself. This section of the chapter further defines intentionality, examines the relationship between intentionality and science, and gives an example of an exercise in intentionality.

In general, the practice of intentionality flows internally from the practice of stillness and meditation described earlier in the chapter. By entering a meditative state and then concentrating on a desired end or communication, events outside oneself may be altered. In other words, the internal energy of the mind may be used to effect changes on external energy or matter. Edgar D. Mitchell (Mitchell & Williams, 1996), a former astronaut educated as an engineer, defines intentionality as follows:

> [T]he active process of desiring or intending an action. Action requires the movement, or transformation, of energy—something each of us does every moment of our lives. Psychoactive people, either naturally or through training, have a greater range of actions they can intentionally and directly initiate with their mind. Psychoactivity is merely a means of managing energy. But if our belief system will not accommodate these natural abilities and they are suppressed early, they will not naturally emerge in the individual; there is just too much dogma in the way. (p. 96)[9]

When the individual enters into a state of harmony through the practice of stillness, the energy of the mind can be harnessed to influence success in goal setting, job seeking, work performance, and other aspects of career, and indeed of life. Useful techniques include visualization, affirmation, and concentration on the energy centers of the body. In visualization, the individual projects himself or herself into the scene in which the desired result is achieved. In carrying out visualizations, the emphasis is on picturing the scene as if it were happening in the present. The more details that can be brought to the scene—of persons, place, objects, colors, sounds, and scents—the more successful the practice is likely to be. In preparing affirmations, the individual again needs to center on the here and now, expressing the belief in the present tense, not the future. Concentrating on the traditional energy centers of the body can provide focus for specific needs. In the ancient Indian system of chakras, seven centers of the body, often pictured as spinning disks, are associated with particular colors, sounds, and life energies. The base chakra, at the bottom of the spine, pictured as red, is associated with material abundance. The second chakra, in the pelvic area, pictured as orange, is associated with sex and its attendant creativity. The third chakra, in the area of the waist, is yellow and is connected to health and personal power. Near the heart is the fourth, green chakra, linked to love. The fifth chakra, which is blue and at the throat, is connected to communication. The sixth and purple chakra is in the forehead, the region of the third eye. It is associated with imagination and insight. The final chakra, at the top of the head, is sometimes pictured as white, the fusion of all the colors. It is tied to spirituality and the universality of the cosmos. Meditating on one or more of the chakras or consciously opening each energy center by breathing in and out the color of the spinning disks can be effective. Finally, intentionality can also be associated with prayer or petition.

It should be noted that in no way is intentionality sufficient by itself. In job seeking, for example, the practice of intentionality is not intended to obviate the need for the rational approaches of networking, job search techniques, writing good résumés, or doing the research for an interview. It does not negate any of those. Intentionality enhances action; intentionality does not supplant action.

Estes (1992) discusses "intentional imagining" after retelling the story of the little match girl, one of the saddest tales of childhood. A poor little girl stands freezing in the cold. She has one match, which she lights. In its glow, she sees the warm home she would like to have. But she stays in the cold and dies in it. Estes contrasts this kind of fantasy, which impedes action, with another, more productive kind of fantasy, which she calls "intentional imaging." She writes,

> This kind of fantasy is like a planning session. It is used as a vehicle to take us forward into action. All successes—psychological, spiritual, financial, and creative—begin with fantasies of this nature. (p. 322)

The passage from Estes suggests that fruitful imagining is a process the individual deliberately chooses rather than a casual mind-drift. It is a way of setting one's mind toward achievement of a goal, a way of finding and identifying the goal. "That the controlling energies of nature are personal, that your own personal thoughts are forces, that the powers of the universe will directly respond to your individual appeals and needs, are propositions which your whole bodily and mental experience will verify" (James, 1902, p. 11).

How can intentionality possibly work? How can one accept an idea that seems so alien to all that is known about the world, to everything that has been learned through the so-called scientific method? There are two approaches to take. The first is to argue that science does not provide the only explanation for the universe. Science, like any other view, was created by fallible humans. Jung (1939/1971) held that argument:

> The conflict between science and religion is in reality a misunderstanding of both. Scientific materialism has merely introduced a new hypostasis, and that is an intellectual sin. It has given another name to the supreme reality and has assumed that this created a new thing and destroyed an old thing. Whether you call the principle of existence "God," "matter," "energy," or anything else you like, you have created nothing; you have simply changed a symbol. (pp. 482–483)

This was also the argument put forth by William James (1902):

> I believe that the claims of the sectarian scientist are, to say the least, premature. The experiences which we have been studying during this hour . . . plainly show the universe to be a more many-sided affair than any sect, even the scientific sect, allows for. What, in the end, are all our verifications but experiences that agree with more or less isolated systems of idea (conceptual systems) that our minds have framed? (p. 120)

In the late twentieth century, many supposedly immutable truths have been thrown into question not by those who simply questioned the truths but by those who have gone beyond doubting the individual beliefs to doubting the very system of thought in which the beliefs were constructed. This has happened in areas of inquiry as varied as literary criticism, educational curriculum revision, census taking, and historiography. "The way in which we divide reality into objects, levels, or any other entities depends largely on our methods of observation. What we see depends on how we look; patterns of matter reflect the patterns of our mind" (Capra, 1988, p. 216).

Indeed, in the world of science, the theory of relativity and subsequent discoveries in the world of physics overturned the previous truth of

Newtonian or classic physics as certainly as Copernicus and Galileo over-threw the belief system of the ancients. And now, support for phenomena such as intentionality and psychoactivity may be coming from the field of physical science itself. Rather than disputing science, one can call upon recent events and findings to garner support for the possibility that inten-tionality actually works in accord with other observable phenomena. There are two principles that underlie current thinking in science and have rele-vance for the consideration of intentionality. Although the principles have arisen from theories and experiments in quantum mechanics, their appli-cation is being explored in other sciences as well. The first principle is con-nectedness; the second is nonlocalness.

Connectedness is easier to explain and more common to human expe-rience. Much of the belief in many religions is based on the belief in con-nections that cannot be seen. Altruistic acts reflect a sense of connection between people who may have no apparent relationship to one another. Synchronicity is offered as an alternative explanation to coincidence when unexpected events that have meaning in one's life occur without seeming cause or effect. Bronowski (1978), in his introduction to a series of lectures to the scientific community, says, "I believe that the world is totally con-nected: that is to say that there are no events anywhere in the universe which are not tied to every other event in the universe" (p. 58).

What evidence is there, however, that an event can influence another indirectly, without linearity and without a chain of cause and effect that can be followed? Chaos theory can explain events in the macroworld (the world in which we humans generally operate and observe). Minuscule changes in circumstance bring about unpredictable outcome behaviors. "Place a cork upstream and it will travel what appears to be a random path. Repeat the experiment, placing the cork as close as humanly possible to the same starting position, and it will follow a completely different trajectory" (Johnson, 1995, p. 92). The behaviors are characterized as nonlinear because the change in the input does not produce an equal change in the output. There is no clear line of relationship between the cause and the effect. The explanation for the seemingly random events of chaotically behaving systems is in strange attractors, which are in themselves mathe-matical equations developed by pattern-seeking human minds. When the equations are plotted or solved, they do not produce lines but complex, often beautiful, patterns, or fractals.

In nonlinearity, then, one sees causal relationships, but the relationships do not make any sense if one looks for a clear one-to-one—or one-to-anything—ratio. Now enter a world even more difficult to fathom, the world of subatomic physics. *Subatomic* means the particles being discussed are smaller than atoms. If you are of a certain age, you were brought up to believe that atoms were the smallest particles; then neutrons and electrons were discovered and they were within atoms. Now even smaller subparticles have been discovered, and they keep getting smaller and smaller—and, as in *Alice in Wonderland*, curiouser and curiouser. It is in the world of subatomic physics, or quantum mechanics, that nonlocalness is observed. By way of definition, localness is the cause and effect of the familiar macroscopic world. If someone wanted to knock a glass off a table, he or she could push it directly, could tilt the table, could push it with a stick, and so on. In any case, a direct relationship between some act (the cause) and the bottle falling (the effect) could be seen. In nonlocalness, scientists can record and observe actual physical phenomena taking place with no known possibility of any agent of any size serving as cause.

Nonlocalness is embedded in the very notion of the now-common expression *quantum leap*. In a quantum leap, a particle vanishes from one place and appears in another at precisely the same time. How is this possible? I haven't a clue. Nor do any of the scientists working today. They can test this and record it with their instruments, but they cannot explain it. At the University of California at Berkeley, photons, the carriers of light, were observed quantum leaping at twice the speed of light. That is, had they actually, physically, crossed the space, they would have done so at twice the speed of light. However, photons are the carriers of light; they cannot move at two times their own speed (Ferris, 1996). How could this happen? No one knows.

There is now an oft-quoted truism that physics has shown that the observer creates the outcome. The actual experiments being so characterized show a world even stranger than that of chaos and quantum leaps. Picture a piece of metal in which there are two holes. Behind the metal is a recording device. Now with my special photon-firing machine, I fire photons at this wall with both holes open. The photons behave in the way that waves behave; that is, they create the kinds of interfering patterns in which the peaks of one wave cancel out the valleys of another as they meet. Waves have this kind of movement. Particles, on the other hand, are bits of things.

They don't have this movement; they have mass. Despite this, if the two holes are open, no matter how many photons are fired, they will behave like waves. This is true even if only one is fired! If one photon is fired, it divides itself, behaves like a wave, and passes through the two holes. If one hole is covered and photons are fired, they behave like particles. Some of them pass through the hole in the wall, just as a bullet would pass through the hole. Some of them hit the wall and fail to pass through, but none of them become waves. Nobody has an explanation for this, but no one denies that it's happening.

At least three possible explanations have been offered by the community of physical scientists for the above observations and for other experiments that demonstrate nonlocalness. First, there is the explanation of hidden variables. That is, there is an explanation but it is not yet known. Second, there are alternate worlds and the particles move among them. And third, time goes both forward and backward. Because time that has passed is still out there somewhere, the particles are able to reenter it. Any or all of these explanations of quantum phenomena may also be explanations of the power and workings of intentionality. Johnson (1995), in a discussion that ranges from the ancient dwellings of the Anasazi to the work at Los Alamos, hypothesizes that information is as real as energy and matter:

> Part Two [of his book, *Fire in the Mind*] will describe an attempt to recast physics and cosmology by climbing back to the trunk of the tree of knowledge (or at least to the base of one of its limbs) and taking a somewhat different branch, in which the seemingly ethereal concept of information is admitted as a fundamental quantity as palpable and real as matter and energy. (p. 7)

I am not the first person to draw analogies between the resonance of the subatomic level and the resonance of expanding consciousness. Edgar D. Mitchell, founder of the Institute of Noetic Sciences, concludes that intentionality works on the same principles as quantum mechanics. He writes,

> A famous mathematical formula, known as Bell's theorem (after its author, the Irish physicist John Bell), holds that the reality of the universe must be non local; in other words, all objects and events in the cosmos are interconnected with one another and respond to one another's change of state. . . . It is this mysterious nonlocality that brings new insight into a number of problems, including those of many enigmatic, subject attributes of consciousness. (Mitchell & Williams, 1996, pp. 109–110)[10]

Intentionality, then, is the act of influencing external states through the mind. That intentionality works has been observed repeatedly both by individuals in the course of their lives and by experiments in parapsychology. An explanation for why intentionality works now seems to be emerging from the domain of science. This section of the chapter concludes with an exercise in intentionality that can be used to develop and enhance interview success in the job search through the use of affirmations.

▼ *Exercise 2*   ***Exercising Intentionality: A Sample Practice***

Sit in a comfortable chair with a firm back or on the floor with your back straight and your legs crossed comfortably. Place your hands on your thighs, palms up and slightly open. Straighten yourself as if you were about to pay attention. Now let your shoulders drop naturally. Breathe slowly, in through your nose and out through your mouth. You may make a sound with your breath as you exhale. Just breathe in and out deeply and evenly for a few moments. Let your breath return to normal. Begin to feel the power of the Earth wherever your body is in contact with the floor or chair. Maintain your contact with the abundant power of the physical, material world. Let the energy of the brown and red Earth, its dryness, its moist fertility enter your body. Keep the Earth's energy within you. At the same time, become aware of the top of your head. Imagine you can feel the electricity of all the spirit in the cosmos. As you draw in one breath, draw in the abundance of the Earth. As you draw in the next, draw in the light of the cosmos. Picture this as you breathe in and out. Any time you lose your concentration in the exercise, just return to your breathing.

Now think of a place that is calm and quiet—a place where you are quite comfortable being alone. Perhaps it is a green meadow near a brook. Maybe it is in a forest as the leaves begin to sprout in early spring or as they begin to turn and fall in autumn. Your safe place may be near a shore where you hear and see the rhythm of the waves. It may be a riverbank. Your safe place may be indoors— a room at your grandparents' house that you loved as a child, or an imaginary room you have dreamed of. There is no one place for all.

Find your safe place. Try to make it as real as you can in your mind's eye. Find the colors in it. Hear the sounds or music or silence. Smell the air. Feel the textures under your feet or in your fingertips. Relax in your safe haven. Spend a few minutes looking around. While you are here, a guide may appear to you. It may be an animal or person, a real figure, a historical one, or someone or something completely imaginary. This is a very safe place for you, and your guide is there only to help you. Your guide will appear only if you need a guide. Your guide cares for you unconditionally.

Relaxed in your safe haven, you are now ready to say six sentences that will affirm your success in coming interviews. If there is a guide, you may want to speak your affirmations to it or her or him. Use the affirmations that follow as they are, modify them, or create your own, as you wish.

Affirmation One: I feel secure in going for the job interview.

Affirmation Two: All my energy will be good for me in the job interview.

Affirmation Three: Everything I say hits just the right note.

Affirmation Four: There is perfect communication between me and the interviewer.

Affirmation Five: The best answers come from me easily and effortlessly.

Affirmation Six: The job that is best for me is mine. ▲

CONCLUSION

There are six implications for counselors and other professionals assisting people in their career development. Each of the implications relies upon an understanding of the three bases developed in this chapter. The first base is the understanding of the nature of meaning in one's lifework and its particular relationship to a sense of connectedness and a sense of absorbedness. The second base is the understanding of how individuals may go about developing their personal sense of meaningfulness and spirituality, using such techniques as meditation and other ways of finding stillness in one's life, of finding the opportunity to reflect without thinking. The third and final base is intentionality, the way of making things happen that will have even greater meaning. What then is the role of the counselor?

The first implication for counselors brings us back to the original idea that each person's life is a work in progress. Accept the process of each client's life and value the opportunity to be allowed into that process.

The second implication reflects the idea that the professional, the helper, herself or himself needs to be in harmony and authentic in relationships. Be open to knowing. Practice knowing through stillness, music, art, poetry to allow yourself to see the relatedness of the universe.

The third implication draws upon the knowledge that the path to harmony and meaningfulness will differ with each individual. Honor the clients' ways of knowing and teach them new ways of knowing. Teach them these methods of stillness, of the use of poetry and art.

The fourth implication for counselors and other professionals is based upon the idea that one is always in a process of learning and that knowledge comes from both the internal world of mindfulness and the external world of experience, from both one's own practice of intentionality and from working with clients or others needing help. Use the knowledge you gain to guide your practice of intentionality.

The fifth implication is based on the idea that many will come to you from traditions other than those with which you are familiar. You will discover that many clients already have practices of spirituality and intentionality. By honoring your clients and familiarizing yourself with their beliefs and practices, you further enable your clients. What you learn from your clients will enhance your own practice as well as give you more to teach to others. Teach the practice of intentionality to your clients in ways that recognize the diversity they bring to you.

Finally, see yourself as a teacher, and follow Krishnamurti's advice:

> When the teacher regards each student as a unique individual, and therefore not to be compared with any other, he is then not concerned with system or method. His sole concern is with "helping" the student to understand the conditioning influences about him and within himself, so that he can face intelligently without fear, the complex process of living, and not add more problems to the already existing mess. (1958/1992b, pp. 27–28)[11]

NOTES

1. From *Zen and the art of motorcycle maintenance: An inquiry into values,* by Robert M. Pirsig, p. 284. Copyright 1974 by Robert M. Pirsig. Reprinted by permission of William Morrow and Co., Inc.

2. From *Zen and the art of motorcycle maintenance: An inquiry into values*, by Robert M. Pirsig, p. 296. Copyright 1974 by Robert M. Pirsig. Reprinted by permission of William Morrow and Co., Inc.

3. Quotations from this section are from *Personal knowledge*, by M. Polanyi, pp. 56–57, 63, and 120. Copyright 1962. Reprinted by permission of the University of Chicago Press.

4. The material in the preceding paragraph was drawn from an earlier article: Bloch, D. P. (1989). *From career information to career knowledge: Self, search, and synthesis. Journal of Career Development, 16,* 119–128.

5. From "What every girl should know, " in *One-half of Robert Davies*, by Robertson Davies, pp. 50–52. Copyright © 1977 by Robertson Davies. Used by permission of Viking Penguin Books USA Inc.

6. From *On right livelihood*, by J. Krishnamurti, p. 86. Copyright © 1992 by the Krishnamurti Foundation Trust Ltd. and the Krishnamurti Foundation of America. Used by permission of HarperCollins Publishers Inc.

7. From *Mind as healer, mind as slayer: A holistic approach to preventing stress disorders*, by K. Pelletier, pp. 225–226. Reprinted by permission of Dell Publishing.

8. The material in the exercises on spirituality and intentionality was drawn from an audiotape series: Bloch, D. P. (1996). *Head and heart to career success* (audiotapes). New York: Self.

9. Reprinted by permission of The Putnam Publishing Group from *The way of the explorer*, by Dr. Edgar D. Mitchell and Dwight Arnan Williams, p. 96. Copyright © 1996 by Dr. Edgar D. Mitchell and Dwight Arnan Williams.

10. Reprinted by permission of The Putnam Publishing Group from *The way of the explorer*, by Dr. Edgar D. Mitchell and Dwight Arnan Williams, pp. 109–110. Copyright © 1996 by Dr. Edgar D. Mitchell and Dwight Arnan Williams.

11. From *On right livelihood*, by J. Krishnamurti, pp. 27–28. Copyright © 1992 by the Krishnamurti Foundation Trust Ltd. and the Krishnamurti Foundation of America. Used by permission of HarperCollins Publishers Inc.

REFERENCES

Bateson, G. (1979). *Mind and nature.* New York: Bantam Books.

Bloch, D. P. (1989). From career information to career knowledge: Self, search, and synthesis. *Journal of Career Development, 16,* pp.119–128.

Bragg, R. (1996, March 5). Big holes where the dignity used to be. *New York Times,* pp. A1, A16–18.

Bridges, W. (1994). *JobShift: How to prosper in a workplace without jobs.* Reading, MA: Addison-Wesley.

Bronowski, J. (1978). *The origins of knowledge and imagination.* New Haven, CT: Yale University Press.

Capra, F. (1988). *Uncommon wisdom: Conversations with remarkable people.* New York: Bantam New Age.

Chopra, D. (1989). *Quantum healing: Exploring the frontiers of mind/body medicine.* New York: Bantam.

Csikszentmihalyi, M. (1990). *Flow: The psychology of optimal experience.* New York: HarperCollins.

Davies, R. (1977). *One half of Robertson Davies.* New York: Penguin.

Estes, C. P. (1992). *Women who run with the wolves: Myths and stories of the wild woman archetype.* New York: Ballantine.

Ferris, T. (1996, September 20). Weirdness makes sense. *New York Times Magazine,* pp. 143–146.

Frost, R. (1949). *Complete poems of Robert Frost.* Austin, TX: Holt, Rinehart, and Winston.

Hall, D. (1993). *Life work*. Boston: Beacon Press.

Handy, C. B. (1989). *Age of unreason*. Boston: Harvard Business School Press.

Holland, J. L. (1992). *Making vocational choices: A theory of vocational personalities and work environments* (2nd ed.). Odessa, FL: Psychological Assessment Resources.

James, W. (1902). *The varieties of religious experience: A study in human nature*. New York: The Modern Library.

Johnson, G. (1995). *Fire in the mind: Science, faith, and the search for order*. New York: Knopf.

Johnson, K. (1996, March 7). In the class of '70, wounded winners. *New York Times*, pp. A1, A20–22.

Jung, C. G. (1971). The difference between Eastern and Western thinking. In J. Campbell (Ed.), *The portable Jung*. (pp. 480–502). New York: Penguin. (Original work published 1939)

Jung, C. G. (1933). *Modern man in search of a soul*. (W. S. Dell & C. F. Baynes, Trans.). Orlando, FL: Harcourt Brace. (Original work published 1931)

Kabat-Zinn, J. (1994). *Wherever you go, there you are: Mindfulness meditation in everyday life*. New York: Hyperion.

Kleinfeld, N. R. (1996, March 4). The company as family, no more. *New York Times*, pp. A1, A12–14.

Kolbert, E., & Clymer, A. (1996, March 8). The politics of layoffs: In search of a message. *New York Times*, pp. A1, A22, A23.

Krishnamurti, J. (1992a). *Commentaries on living first series*, Chapter 88. In J. Krishnamurti, *On right livelihood*. San Francisco: Harper San Francisco. (Original work published 1956)

Krishnamurti, J. (1992b). *Commentaries on living second series*, Chapter 31. In J. Krishnamurti, *On right livelihood*. San Francisco: Harper San Francisco. (Original work published 1958)

Krishnamurti, J. (1992c). *On education*, Chapter 8. In J. Krishnamurti, *On right livelihood*. San Francisco: Harper San Francisco. (Original work published 1974)

Krumboltz, J. D., & Mitchell, A. M. (1990). Social learning approach to career decision making: In D. Brown & L. Brooks (Eds.), *Career choice and development* (2nd ed.) (pp. 145–196). San Francisco: Jossey-Bass.

Krumboltz, J. D., Mitchell, A. M., & Jones, G. B. (1976). A social learning theory of career selection. *Counseling Psychologist, 6*, pp. 71–81.

Lao Tsu. (1989). *Tao Te Ching*. (G. F. Feng & J. English, Trans.). New York: Vintage Books.

Lewin, K. (1935). *A dynamic theory of personality: Selected papers*. New York: McGraw-Hill.

Mitchell, E., & Williams, D. (1996). *The way of the explorer: An Apollo astronaut's journey through the material and mystical worlds*. New York: Putnam.

Parsons, F. (1909). *Choosing a vocation*. Boston: Houghton Mifflin.

Pelletier, K. R. (1977). *Mind as healer, mind as slayer: A holistic approach to preventing stress disorders*. New York: Dell.

Pirsig, R. M. (1984). *Zen and the art of motorcycle maintenance: An inquiry into values*. New York: Morrow.

Polanyi, M. (1962). *Personal knowledge: Toward a post-critical philosophy.* Chicago: University of Chicago Press.

Rifkin, J. (1995). The end of work: The decline of the global labor force and the dawn of the post-market era. New York: Putnam.

Rimer, S. (1996, March 6). A hometown feels less like home. *New York Times,* pp. A1, A16–18.

Sanger, D. E., & Lohr, S. (1996, March 9). A search for answers to avoid the lay-offs. *New York Times,* pp. A1, A12–13.

Savickas, M. L, & Walsh, W. B. (Eds.). (1996). *Handbook of career counseling theory and practice.* Palo Alto, CA: Davies-Black.

Sciolino, E. (1996, October 27). Senators retire, one to marry, some to write. *New York Times,* pp. A1, A11.

Super, D. (1990). A life span, life space approach to career development. In D. Brown & L. Brooks (Eds.), *Career choice and development* (2nd ed.) (pp. 197–261). San Francisco: Jossey-Bass.

Super, D. (1994). A life span, life space perspective on convergence. In M. L. Savickas & R. Lent (Eds.), *Convergence in career development theories: Implications for science and practice* (pp. 63–74). Palo Alto, CA: Consulting Psychologists Press.

Uchitelle, L., & Kleinfeld, N. R. (1996, March 3). On the battlefields of business, millions of casualties. *New York Times,* pp. A1, A26–29.

Ueland, B. (1987). *If you want to write: A book about art, independence, and spirit* (2nd ed.). St. Paul, MN: Graywolf Press.

Zane, J. P. (1996, May 26). Doublespeak. *New York Times,* p. D7.

CHAPTER TEN

Spirituality and Career Assessment

Metaphors and Measurement

Lee J. Richmond
Loyola College

I N NEMIROV, a small town in eastern Europe not unlike the town where the now famous Tevye of *Fiddler on the Roof* fame lived, a story is told of a Chassidic rabbi, his devoted flock, and a skeptic. The people, of course, were very, very poor, the rabbi very, very holy, and the skeptic very, very unbelieving. The story is as follows: The people believed that each year, just prior to the Penitential Season marking the Days of Awe that began the Jewish New Year, their rabbi went to heaven. After all, the Jews, however poor, still needed to eke out some kind of a livelihood, even as they needed good health and good matches for their sons and daughters, and they believed that their rabbi went to heaven to intercede on their behalf. One day, a skeptic, a Jewish shoemaker from Lithuania, arrived in town, and on that day the Jews of the town were very happy because sometime within the next twenty-four hours their rabbi was going to heaven, they said, to plead for them before the Throne of the Most High.

The skeptic called them foolish Jews for believing this. Not even Moses ascended to heaven, let alone a poor rabbi. Nevertheless, the skeptic was intrigued, so he decided to follow the rabbi, even to hide in the rabbi's house so that he would be able to see everything the rabbi did that day and thereby discredit the notions of the rabbi's foolish flock.

That evening, when the Jews of Nemirov journeyed to the river to symbolically rid themselves of their sins, their rabbi was not among them, nor was he in the house of prayer. "He must be in heaven," a congregant announced, and all of the others agreed.

Meanwhile the skeptic, hiding under the rabbi's bed, saw the rabbi dress himself in the clothing of a Polish peasant. On his feet he placed high boots, and on his head a woodsman's cap, and on his body a greatcoat. The rabbi then placed a sack in the inner pocket of the coat and tied a large leather belt about his waist. The skeptic could not imagine what was going on until the rabbi took hold of an axe. "For sure," thought the skeptic, "the rabbi knows I'm here and he is going to kill me."

Instead the rabbi put the axe in his belt, exited his small house, and walked deep into the woods. The skeptic followed and watched the rabbi fell a tree, chop it into logs, and then chop some of the logs more finely into sticks. The rabbi then bundled the wood and placed it into the large sack, which he took from his greatcoat. He then dragged the sack of wood even more deeply into the forest to a small hut where a poor widow lived.

The rabbi knocked on the door. "Who is there?" cried the widow. "It is Ivan," said the rabbi, "Ivan the woodcutter. I have heard that you are ill, and it is very cold, so I have brought you some wood." The woman opened the door and, from behind the tree where he was hiding, the skeptic heard the woman say, "I have no money to pay for wood." She coughed. "My son is looking for work in the next town, but he has found none," she said. The rabbi, alias Ivan, said, "He will find work soon; then you will pay. Plenty of time." The rabbi then entered the widow's hut. Through the window, the skeptic saw him light a fire, give the woman a crust of bread from his pocket, and then exit the house.

At daybreak, when the Jews were going to synagogue for morning prayers, they once again encountered the skeptic. "Well," one said to him, "our beloved rabbi went to heaven last night. Next year will surely be a little better for us. But you don't believe us, do you?" he asked.

Quietly the skeptic said, "Yes, I do. He went to heaven, if not higher. In fact, I saw him do it."

This story is an adaptation of a story told by the Yiddish writer I. L. Peretz.[1] I heard it for the first time as a young child, and I guess I never totally forgot it, although it was relegated to a level below my consciousness for years. However, when I began to think about spirituality and career assessment, I strangely enough recalled the story. It seemed to illustrate the whole notion of career assessment. What one sees and how one sees it depend to a large extent on who is doing the looking and what he or she is looking for—on the mindset of the one who does the looking as much as on objective measures.

If each of us were born with a built-in omniscient observer system, one that could monitor and register our personality characteristics, our interests, and our abilities while at the same time monitor the seen and unseen universe in which we live, and if this system could funnel all it detected through the prism of our individual aspirations and values, formal career assessment would not be necessary. However, no such inner guidance system exists. Therefore people use instruments to assist them toward their individual career destinations. The career journey is by nature a spiritual journey insofar as meaningful work in life links who we are as individuals to the society in which we live. Ultimately it also links our world to both the worlds of our ancestors and the worlds of our children.

The instruments we use are not mindless. Each is based on a theory—a set of ideas that exists in the consciousness of the instrument maker. These ideas relate to the nature of human personality and to how human beings live in the world. The purpose of this chapter is to link theory to practice in career assessment and to demonstrate that the course people steer in order to discover self in the work world is a spiritual journey not unlike the journey taken by the rabbi of Nemirov when he reached the highest heaven while chopping wood and delivering it to one in need. It is in fact a journey into meaning.

THE NATURE OF WORK AND ITS LINK TO SPIRITUALITY

There are many definitions of work. These definitions range from labor, the exertion of physical strength or mental effort in order to perform a task or duty, to the transference of energy, the performance of service, and ultimately to artistic creation and the performance of religious acts (Merriam-Webster, 1993). The word *career*, which originally meant a road or a street, has come to mean a course, a passage, a charge, or an encounter. A career is a pursuit of achievement or something that is taken as a permanent calling (Merriam-Webster, 1993). Although the word *work* and the word *career* are often used interchangeably, as such they have most frequently been used in the context of job or occupation. Only recently has career been defined as all the roles one plays (Super, 1984), or as one's life (Miller-Tiedeman, 1989).

However, if one accepts the definition of career as a journey that one feels called or commissioned to take on his or her road through life, and work as the energy one expends along the way in the performance of labor, service, and acts of creation, one cannot escape the fact that spirituality permeates work. In a wonderful book entitled *The Reinvention of Work,* Fox (1995) asserts that there is only one work going on in the universe—the "Great Work" of creation itself—"the work of creation unfolding, the work of evolution or creativity in the universe" (p. 61). And we, according to Fox, in whatever profession or occupation we may find ourselves, are each and all a part of this creation. Because human work is a part of the ongoing work of the universe, Fox suggests that people must commit to the inner work that at this juncture in history we so desperately need, so that, as Fox states, "our inner work can feed our outer work . . . in authentic creation" (p. 297). For Fox, work has sacramental implications. To this end, he developed a *Spirituality and Work Questionnaire* (found in the epilogue of his book) in which questions relate to joy in work. He asks, "Do I experience joy in work, and do others experience it as a result of my work? Do I experience awe and wonder through it? And will it be a blessing for generations to come?" In connecting human work to the "Great Work" of the ongoing creation of the universe, work is more than job. It concerns not only what we do but also how we do it and how we view it.

There are other measures of spirituality that relate to work. These instruments generally measure holistic wellness. Recently, Witmer, Sweeney, and Myers completed the development of the WEL Inventory, which is designed to help individuals identify their current level of wellness, assess personal resources for wellness, and develop a plan for living life more fully. The instrument is predicated on a model originally developed by Witmer and Sweeney (1992) based upon research across several disciplines and spanning more than four decades. The model asserts that there are five basic tasks in life: (1) spirituality, (2) self-regulation, (3) work, recreation, and leisure, (4) friendship, and (5) love. The five tasks of the model extend to sixteen dimensions that are measured by the instrument. They are as follows:

1. Spirituality
2. Sense of worth
3. Sense of control
4. Realistic beliefs
5. Emotional responsibility and management
6. Intellectual stimulation, problem solving, creativity
7. Sense of humor
8. Nutrition
9. Exercise
10. Self care
11. Stress management
12. Gender identity
13. Cultural identity
14. Work, recreation, and leisure
15. Friendship
16. Love

The instrument operationally defines each of these dimensions. The spiritual dimension, for instance, relates to the existence of a power greater than self, the sense of being connected to it, and the awe and wonder that flows from that perceived relationship. The work, recreation, and leisure dimension relates to having job or leisure satisfaction and adequate financial security, and achieving rest and renewal from leisure time activities.

The WEL Inventory is a pencil-and-paper instrument on which test takers rank more than 100 items on a five-point scale ranging from *strongly agree* to *strongly disagree*. It yields a total wellness and a perceived wellness score. Part of the beauty of the instrument is that it causes a person to think about how spirituality, coupled with self-direction in work and leisure and in friendship and love, radiates outward and influences global events through business and industry, media, government, community, family, religion, and education, as shown in Figure 2 on page 214.

Another less formal inventory that connects spirituality to work through discernment of one's own personal theology is contained in the book *Seeds of Sensitivity* (Wicks, 1995). This inventory consists of a series of questions. The questions begin by asking for clarification of one's own image of God,

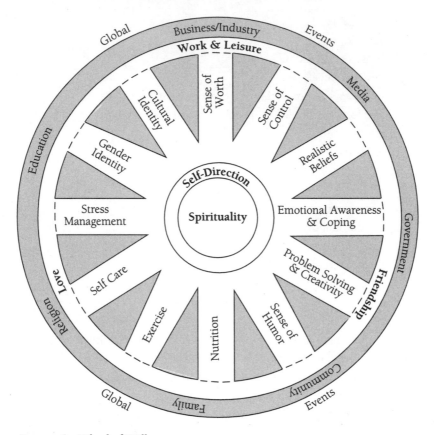

Figure 2   Wheel of Wellness

Note: Copyright 1996 J. Melvin Witmer, Thomas J. Sweeney, & Jane E. Myers. Reprinted with permission.

lead to one's relationship with that image, and end with one's image of God and one's relationship with God as these affect difficult relationships with friends, family, and colleagues. This inventory also causes one to examine one's image of God and one's relationship with God in accordance with one's ideals and fears and one's work and leisure. Wicks (1995) also offers a psychological health checklist in which there are eight categories with questions related to each. The checklist, seen in Figure 3, contains additional items. As Wicks states, "All of the questions are designed to encourage personal responsibility" (p. 130).

In their *Inventory of Spirituality*, Rayburn and Richmond (1996) link spirituality with a sense of connectedness, both to the universe and to others. This twenty-seven-item pencil-and-paper test asks the degree to which

1. **Attention to physical health:** Rest, diet, and activity—leisure and work are elements that rely on our attitude; are we balancing them?
2. **Assertiveness:** Are we aware of our feelings and beliefs, and do we present them to others in a timely, appropriate fashion?
3. **Values and meaning:** Are we aware of ethics in how we live? Do our actions reflect what we believe and value?
4. **Self-awareness:** Do we have times when we look at our thoughts, feelings, and behavior in a curious and constructive fashion?
5. **Acceptance of love and criticism:** Are we willing to accept rather than devalue the love around us? Are we willing to accept criticism rather than project blame or be hypersensitive?
6. **Creative ways of relating to others:** When our primary style isn't working well, are we willing to entertain varying approaches such as being more direct, having greater patience, standing aside, confronting, accepting?
7. **"Soft power":** Are we willing to see and act upon the value of gentleness, imagination, active listening, relaxation, and patience?
8. **Cognition:** Do we take the time to plan, prioritize, and get clarity on issues?

FIGURE 3   Psychological Health Checklist

Note: Excerpted from *Seeds of Sensitivity* by Robert J. Wicks. Copyright 1995 by Ava Maria Press, Notre Dame, IN 46556. Used with permission of the publisher.

persons regard their work as a means of enriching the lives of others. It was by taking responsibility for self, exerting self-direction, and enriching the life of another soul that the rabbi of Nemirov connected Earth to heaven. Perhaps we can do the same.

CAREER DEVELOPMENT AND PERSONALITY: THEORY-BASED ASSESSMENT

Since the time of Freud, the ability to love and to work, and perhaps to play, has been considered the hallmark of a healthy personality. This is because both love and work imply connectedness. The opposite of connectedness is isolation, resulting in loneliness. Loneliness, the subjective experience of being *separated* from one's fellow human beings, is a psychological problem of epic proportions. But how does one avoid loneliness and acquire a sense of connectedness to other human beings through work? Or, better asked, how does one connect to one's inner self and really get to know it, so that in turn one can connect one's inner self—one's personality, interests, and abilities—to the outer world of work, leisure, and community? It is here that theories of personality come into play.

Two members of Freud's original group, Jung and Adler, each developed theories that link personality to work, and these theories have aided in development of both formal and informal assessment tools. One such tool is the *Myers-Briggs Type Indicator®* personality inventory, known as the MBTI. The MBTI is today's most commonly used instrument when assessing personality type. Developed by Katharine Briggs and Isabel Briggs-Myers, the MBTI is based on attempts to explain individual differences according to a typology of the psyche attributed to the Swiss psychiatrist Jung. Jung based his personality theory on the assumption that the psyche (or mind) has both a conscious and an unconscious level, the latter being comprised of both a personal unconscious and a collective unconscious. Also significant is that a person possesses a persona, a mask that he or she wears outwardly and shows to the world, and a shadow, the archetype of darkness that represents the features of personality that one wishes to hide from others and from self. Reconciliation of opposites occupies a large place in Jungian thinking, and it is against that backdrop that Jung's typology of the psyche is understood. Jung (1933) postulates two basic attitudes, or inclinations, to act or react in a certain direction. The two basic attitudes are introversion and extroversion. Jung insists that each person possesses both an introverted and extroverted attitude. If introversion is conscious, then extroversion is unconscious, and vice versa. In Jungian psychology, introversion is energy oriented toward the inner world of individual perception, fantasy, and dreams. Extroversion, in contrast, is characterized by the turning of energy outward toward the external, objective world.

Jung also postulates four functions—thinking, feeling, sensation, and intuition. Each of the functions, according to Jung, can be extroverted or introverted, depending on a person's basic attitude. Jung claims that the function of thinking is something like judging on the basis of rationality, whereas the feeling function bases judgment primarily on values. He sees intuition and sensation as perceptive functions as opposed to rational ones. To Jung, sensation signifies a person's reception of information obtained through the senses, whereas intuition is more creative and more rudimentary.

Jung formed his concepts of psychic functions from the notions expressed in current speech (Jung, 1933). He said, "I took thinking as it

TABLE 1   The 16 MBTI Types

ISTP	ISFJ	INFJ	INTJ
ISTP	ISFP	INFP	INTP
ESTP	ESFP	ENFP	ENTP
ESTJ	ESFJ	ENFJ	ENTJ

was generally understood because I was struck by the fact that some people do more of it than others" (p. 89). Jung therefore claims that whereas philosophers might argue over his terminology, it is quite clear to the common person.

Nevertheless the MBTI attempts to clean up Jung's act. It speaks of preference pairs: Extraversion (E) and Introversion (I) (life attitudes); Sensing (S) and Intuition (N) (perceiving functions); Thinking (T) and Feeling (F) (judging functions); and Judging (J) and Perceiving (P) (life orientation). The combinations of these types break out into the sixteen MBTI personality types as seen in Table 1.

Each of these types is a tool for understanding one's own type and the differences between it and other types.

The MBTI instrument is widely used. Human resources personnel use it for team building in business and industry. Career advisers search its manual for how many of what type of people are in which occupations. Teachers explain how gifts differ, and even couples in marriage counseling use it to create glimpses into areas of compatibility and incompatibility. Jung (1933), however, sees his theory of types as a part of historical progression in the human being's attempt to understand self. "Since earliest times," he writes, "attempts have been made to classify individuals according to type and thus bring order to confusion" (pp. 82–83). Astrology attempted to do this. So did Greek physicians who described four dispositions or types—phlegmatic, sanguine, choleric, and melancholic. Jung sees his method as more scientific than these and as a road to self-discovery, which he views as a spiritual journey. Speaking of this, Jung writes, "The manifestations of spirit are truly wondrous, and as varied as creation itself" (p. 224).

Completing the MBTI inventory and seriously reflecting on one's type is one way of connecting with self. Through proper use of the instrument, a person can find his or her preferred functions: the dominant and auxiliary. One can also discern the two less-preferred functions: the tertiary and the inferior. The less-preferred functions are hidden deeply in the unconscious. On the MBTI tool, they are opposite the dominant and auxiliary. By knowing this, one can view one's shadow side and see it as an opportunity for spiritual growth and career challenge.

Jung's theory is not the only way by which one can view personality. Adler (1956) had other ideas that led to other means of assessing it. He thought that all psychological phenomena are unified within the individual in a self-consistent manner. Therefore the individual strives for a goal, and his or her behavior is directed by his or her beliefs about final purpose. One acts on what one believes to be true. People are motivated in the present by their perceptions of the future. Adler's criteria for measuring psychological health is social interest. He refers to it as the "barometer of normality," the instrument by which the standard of a life could be measured. Adler (1979) further claims that people strive for superiority and for success not only for themselves but also for all humankind.

According to Adler (1956), each of us develops a style of life that can be discerned through early recollections. If style of life changes, early recollections change. Several activities based on Adlerian theory can be used as assessment tools to help one understand one's personality and link personality to career development and occupational choice. One such activity is to remember and name a favorite childhood toy and remember the activities engaged in while playing with that toy or game.

One person who completed this activity remembered playing with a magnifying glass and a cloak. She would don the cloak and walk in the alley behind her home in the city seeking clues to resolve an imagined mystery. She extracted discarded letters from trash cans and although she could not yet read she pretended to decode secret messages. Today she is a forensic psychologist using clues found in tests and drawings to reconstruct a lifestyle and solve mysteries for the court system. Hardly standardized, a thorough examination of the play that one enjoyed as a child can nevertheless be a powerful assessment tool when linking personality to the work world of adulthood.

Another assessment activity related to early recollections and a final goal is the drawing of a tree. An individual is told to draw a tree that is representative of his or her life, then add the sun, rain, and any other elements that helped the tree to grow. Lastly the individual is told to pay attention to the foliage and to any fruit the tree might bear, and to also draw these into the picture. Then the individual is again informed that the tree is a metaphor for life and that the tree should be examined in that light by supplying answers to the following questions:

1. In what kind of soil was the tree planted? Are its roots deep or shallow?
2. In what kind of soil did the tree grow?
3. Was the tree ever transplanted when it was young? Older? If so, did the soil change? What happened to the tree then?
4. Who nourished the tree in its youth? And who nourishes it now?
5. What kind of nourishment did the tree receive in its youth, and what kind of nourishment does it need now?
6. Did the tree receive what it needed in its youth? And is it receiving what it needs now?
7. Does the tree have fruit? What kind? And are the fruits plentiful and pleasing?
8. Does the tree want to bear different fruits? If so, name them.
9. What does the tree need by way of supportive soil and nourishment to bear more fruit or new fruit?
10. Describe the tree. Is it sturdy? Flexible? And if it has to be transplanted now, how could it best survive?

Of course, the person who answers the questions answers as a person, not as a tree. The exercise is profound. Some people are as sturdy as oaks and would like to be as flexible as willows. Some see themselves bearing many fruits (talents, abilities, and gifts). Others see themselves with few fruits or none; still others are planted in sand, and their roots struggle to survive. Some cannot get to water and parch as brush in the desert.

This exercise has been proven so intense that counselors who lead groups and who make this a group draw-and-share exercise often require more than two hours of processing time for a group of six to eight persons. Of course, what is being asked for are early life recollections and future goals, as these are lived out in social context. The metaphor, however, links mind to emotion and past to future in the unity of the human personality. As such, the activity is directly linked to Adler's personality theory.

INTERESTS AND ABILITIES:
THEORY-BASED ASSESSMENTS

In addition to the major philosophical questions regarding personality—
From where do I come? To where do I go? Who am I as a person?—there
are questions career seekers ask that demand immediate and practical
answers. These questions relate to interests and abilities. What are my
interests? What is my knowledge? What are my skills? Furthermore, if
work is to be meaningful, then interests, knowledge, and skills must pass
through the funnel of values. Values are the ultimate determiners of choice,
as seen in Figure 4.

Perhaps nothing is more closely related to joy or at least satisfaction
with one's work than one's interest in it. The theorist most closely associated with the measurement of interests is John Holland, creator of many
instruments, the best known of which is the *Self-Directed Search*, or SDS. A
scholar in the area of personality as it relates to interests and of interests as
they relate to the workplace, Holland (1973, 1985) developed a typology
of people and of occupational environments that allows prediction of sat-
isfactory outcome in occupational selection on the basis of closeness of fit.
Holland's theory is summarized in seven principal elements: (1) Most people can be characterized as one of these six personality types: Realistic,
Investigative, Artistic, Social, Enterprising, or Conventional, as seen in
Table 2 and Figure 5. (2) There are six kinds of working environments:
Realistic (R), Investigative (I), Artistic (A), Social (S), Enterprising (E), and
Conventional (C). Each environment is dominated by a given type of personality. (3) People search for environments that will let them exercise
skills and abilities, express their attitudes and values, and take on agreeable
problems and roles. For example, realistic people seek realistic environments. (4) A person's behavior is determined by an interaction between his
or her personality and the characteristics of the work environment. (5) The
degree of congruence between a person and an occupational environment
can be estimated by using a hexagonal model as seen in Figure 5. (6) The
degree of consistency within a person or environment is also defined using
the hexagonal model. Adjacent types on the hexagon are the most consistent. (7) The degree of differentiation of a person or an environment mod-
ifies predictions made from a person's SDS profile, from an occupational
code, or from the action between the two. Some persons or environments

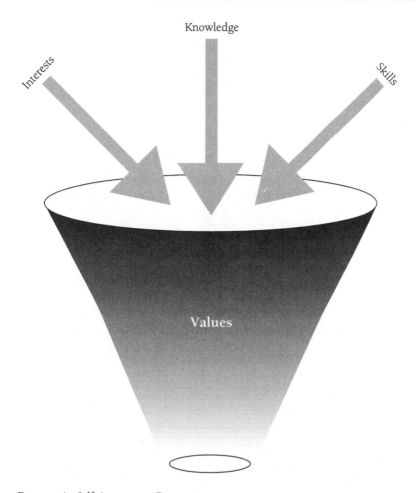

FIGURE 4 Self-Assessment Process
Note: Used with the permission of Linda K. Kemp.

are more clearly defined than others (Holland, Powell, & Fritzsche, 1994, pp. 5–7).

Holland's theory seems simple, and yet it is profound. Interests reflect what one likes to do in both work and leisure. If one can identify them by using the SDS, or any other instrument, one is a step ahead in knowing what jobs (and what leisure activities) one is likely to enjoy.

One might think, however, that interests are obvious. It seems almost silly to have to take a test to know what they are. But the fact is that

TABLE 2   Holland's Six Personality Types

The **Realistic** type likes realistic jobs such as automobile mechanic, aircraft controller, surveyor, farmer, electrician. Has mechanical abilities, but may lack social skills. Is described as:

Asocial	Inflexible	Practical
Conforming	Materialistic	Self-effacing
Frank	Natural	Thrifty
Genuine	Normal	Uninsightful
Hardheaded	Persistent	Uninvolved

The **Investigative** type likes investigative jobs such as biologist, chemist, physicist, anthropologist, geologist, medical technologist. Has mathematical and scientific ability but often lacks leadership ability. Is described as:

Analytical	Independent	Rational
Cautious	Intellectual	Reserved
Complex	Introspective	Retiring
Critical	Pessimistic	Unassuming
Curious	Precise	Unpopular

The **Artistic** type likes artistic jobs such as composer, musician, stage director, writer, interior decorator, actor/actress. Has artistic abilities— writing, musical, or artistic—but often lacks clerical skills. Is described as:

Complicated	Imaginative	Intuitive
Disorderly	Impractical	Nonconforming
Emotional	Impulsive	Open
Expressive	Independent	Original
Idealistic	Introspective	Sensitive

although a person may know something about what he or she likes to do, one's thoughts are often piecemeal and not easily related to the world of work activity. The beauty of the Holland theory is that it organizes data about interests in such a way that it relates interests to personality and through personality to occupations. Interest tests frequently offer lists of activities and ask people to state whether they like them or dislike them. The tests then organize the data according to some theoretically based schematic. If they are tests using the theory or schematic of Holland (RIASEC), the results are a three-digit Holland code, such as SAE or IRC, or any other combination of the six types. The code describes personality through traits that correspond to occupational characteristics. For instance, the Social, Artistic, and Enterprising type would tend to like such professions as counselor or teacher, whereas the IRC type would be more likely to enjoy some engineering options or perhaps radioscopy.

TABLE 2   Holland's Six Personality Types (continued)

The **Social** type likes social jobs such as teacher, religious worker, counselor, clinical psychologist, psychiatric case worker, speech therapist. Has social skills and talents but often lacks mechanical and scientific ability. Is described as:

Ascendant	Helpful	Responsible
Cooperative	Idealistic	Sociable
Empathetic	Kind	Tactful
Friendly	Patient	Understanding
Generous	Persuasive	Warm

The **Enterprising** type likes enterprising jobs such as salesperson, manager, business executive, television producer, sports promoter, buyer. Has leadership and speaking abilities but often lacks scientific ability. Is described as:

Acquisitive	Energetic	Flirtatious
Adventurous	Excitement-	Optimistic
Agreeable	seeking	Self-confident
Ambitious	Exhibitionistic	Sociable
Domineering	Extroverted	Talkative

The **Conventional** type likes conventional jobs such as bookkeeper, stenographer, financial analyst, banker, cost estimator, tax expert. Has clerical and arithemetic ability but often lacks artistic abilities. Is described as:

Careful	Inflexible	Persistent
Conforming	Inhibited	Practical
Conscientious	Methodical	Prudish
Defensive	Obedient	Thrifty
Efficient	Orderly	Unimaginative

Is there a way of obtaining a Holland code without taking a formal test? Holland himself seems to think so. He contends that if a person can list ten occupational daydreams and then seek each occupational daydream in *The Occupation Finder* (Holland, 1989), a booklet published to accompany the SDS that organizes occupations according to RIASEC, the sum total of the codes for the daydreams would approximate the code the person would receive if he or she took the SDS. In fact, Holland lists this activity in the SDS test booklet (1990, p. 3). It is not scored with the inventory, but it allows the test taker to compare his or her daydream code with the inventory code. Most often, the two codes are the same.

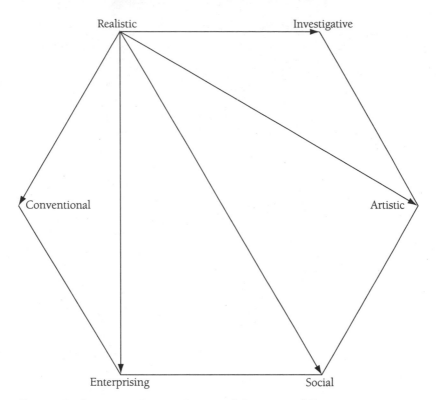

FIGURE 5   Congruence Between Person and Occupational Environment

Richard Bolles, author of *What Color Is Your Parachute?*, developed a game called "The Party" (1997, p. 80) that allows a person to discover his or her Holland code. The game is widely used. One business that uses it is the United States Postal Service; their human resources personnel train managers to understand the relationship between interests and the world of work. They do this by asking participants to pretend they are at a party. The participants are told that it is a large party and many postal people who they don't know are there. These people are in groups, talking to one another. Together the groups form a configuration that looks like a hexagon, shown in Figure 6. At one location, the upper left, there are people who are athletic, who like doing mechanical work or outside work. At another location, moving clockwise, are those who like to investigate, analyze, and solve problems. Separate but not too far away are those who are

With which group of people do you best fit?

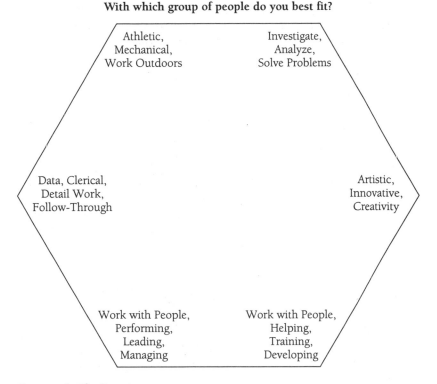

FIGURE 6   The Party
Note: © Richard Bolles. Used with permission.

artistic, innovative, and like to do creative things. At yet another point are people who work with people, helping, training, and developing. Then there is a group of those who work with people as executives and managers. At the last location, there are those who like clerical, data, and detail work. Manager trainees are then asked which group they would gravitate toward first, then second, and then third. The three combinations from first to last would constitute their Holland code and illustrate their primary interests.

Interests are clearly an important part of self-assessment, but of equal importance is ability. Ability consists of knowledge and skills. Skills can be defined as those things that a person is capable of doing. One can have skills in several interest areas. Skills may exist as a result of talent, but they can also be acquired through training. Whether innate or acquired, skills can be enhanced through further education or practice. Whether one chooses to enhance skills in any given area depends on many factors.

Usually enhancing a skill involves some sacrifice of time, money, or relationships. What one chooses to sacrifice or whether one chooses to sacrifice at all depend upon one's personal circumstances and the value one places on the skill.

Knowledge is different from skill in that it involves perceiving directly and having an awareness and understanding of what is known. Knowledge is gained through association and experience and usually involves the acquisition of information through learning. It is not innate, though the intelligence used to acquire knowledge is; nor does knowledge necessarily involve doing. Skills are separate from knowledge in that they imply the ability to use knowledge. It is interesting that the Hebrew scriptures make this distinction. In Scripture, when given the law, the Hebrew people were told to hear (know) and do (act).

The *Dictionary of Occupational Titles* (U.S. Department of Labor, 1991) divides the skills and knowledge needed for occupations into three categories: data, people, and things. The category of *data* involves the ability to compare, copy, compute, compile, analyze, coordinate, and synthesize. The category called *people* involves the ability to take instructions, serve, speak and signal, divert, supervise, instruct, and mentor. The category called *things* involves the ability to handle, feed (as into machinery), tend, manipulate, operate or control, do precision work, and set up. All abilities are listed from those requiring the least skill to those requiring the most. All occupations are listed not only by title but also by degree of skill required in each of the three areas: data, people, and things.

There are many measures of ability relative to skills and to interests. These tests are called achievement and/or aptitude tests and they are legion. Schoolchildren take them routinely. Adults take them at will. Such tests are often given as part of the job acquisition process.

But even when skills, knowledge, ability, and interests are identified, meaningful work does not necessarily flow. All assessment information must be seen in the light of values if work is to have meaning. It stands to reason that one would obtain greater satisfaction from a position compatible with one's interests and abilities than from an incompatible one. Nevertheless, a person with an SAE Holland code who has the ability to instruct and mentor and an inclination to teach might not enjoy that teaching position if he or she were teaching for an organization whose values were inherently different from his or her own. Nor would one necessarily accept a promotion, with personality-compatible duties and high pay, if such a promotion involved a move away from a beloved family member who happened to be terminally ill. Values are the prism through which all self-assessment information passes, and they are the filter through which all decisions are crystallized. Values can anchor persons in place or move them to the ends of the Earth. Values can be measured by formal means. They can also be discerned informally. One informal group method is the values auction: Participants imagine they are at an auction. Everyone at the auction is given a descriptive brochure of items to be sold. Participants are also given a budget worksheet with the items to be auctioned listed on it, as seen in Figure 7. Participants are asked to prioritize the items they feel are important for them to have. Then, out of an allotted amount of "money" given them to spend, participants are told to allocate portions of it to significant items. They cannot exceed their allocation. A mock auction is held. On the budget worksheet, participants list what they budgeted, what they spent, and funds remaining. From this activity they learn what is valuable. They also learn what they will sacrifice for that which is most valuable. Some people never get anything; they are overcautious or con- fused about values. Often this simulation approximates their behavior and condition in life.

There are many standardized tests of values. Most of these tests are based on the test maker's theory of values. Schein (1990) developed an instrument entitled the Career Orientation Inventory, based on a values concept that he called *Career Anchors*. The values, or *anchors,* according to Schein, are technical/functional competence, general managerial compe- tence, security/stability, entrepreneurial creativity, autonomy/indepen- dence, service/dedication to a cause, pure challenge, and lifestyle. The strongest values are those anchors that keep people in place, those that people are least likely to pull up.

The marketplace offers checklists of personal values, interpersonal val- ues, and work values. Some are standardized; others are not. However, one comes to know one's values; they are integrally connected to meaning in life. Values do change over time, but Frankle (1963), the existential psy- chiatrist who is credited with creating logotherapy, sees human beings as responsible for the fulfillment of values and the creation of meaning in their lives. Frankle speaks of three kinds of values: (1) creative values, which one exercises through productive work; (2) experiential values,

Directions: Prioritize the items you feel are most significant to you. Number them in order of importance, 1 being the highest. Then place the amount you are willing to spend on each item. Remember not to exceed $500 total.

Keep a tally on how much you actually spent for each item (even if it's only one item) and at the conclusion of the auction place the funds you have remaining in the last column.

Auction Item	Priority	$500 Budget	Spent	Remaining Funds
Adventure				
Culture				
Family				
Freedom				
Health				
Helping Others				
High Income				
Independence				
Leadership				
Leisure				
Love				
Nature				
Prestige				
Productivity				
Religion				
Security				
Success				
Variety				

FIGURE 7   Value Auction Budget Worksheet

Note: Used with the permission of Linda K. Kemp.

known through enjoyment of the good and the beautiful in life; and (3) attitudinal values, which can exist even when other values are not to be found. Attitudinal values can be experienced even in death camps. They involve giving unique meaning to life, even in the face of suffering and dying. Frankle created a term, *nöogenic neuroses,* to describe the sickness that comes from a loss of values, a loss of a sense of meaning in life. Some say that loss of sense of meaning is the neurosis of our time.

The rabbi of Nemirov had strong values and a sense of meaning in life. It was rooted in service. He had the ability to both hear and do. He was certainly concerned about people, and he was also enterprising. He had the skill not only to teach his congregants but also to cut and haul wood and build a fire. Though he was himself poor, he was able to share his bread with a sick woman. His attitude was that life is precious and to save a life is a prayer. His focus was so direct and so singular that he enlightened a skeptic, and the skeptic too climbed higher.

ASSESSING LIFE-AS-CAREER

Like interests, abilities, and values, our notions of career itself can and do change over time. Recently several career theorists have begun to talk about career as life. Just as Fox (1955) linked human work to the great work of the universe, Super began to look at career as distinct from occupation. He created the Life Career Rainbow (Super, 1990) to suggest that in addition to the worker role, people play eight other roles in life: child, student, leisurite, citizen, spouse, homemaker, parent, and pensioner. These roles are played in the home, community, school, and workplace, with each role predominantly played in one theater. Roles are often played simultaneously, and it is the sequential combination of roles that comprises one's lifestyle. One's lifestyle is lived in a structure that Super calls one's life space. A person's career pattern is the combination of life cycle and life space. Super portrays this as a Life Career Rainbow, shown in Figure 8.

The Life Career Rainbow can be used as an assessment device. One can look at it and answer questions such as the following: What roles am I playing now? Which have I played in the past? What roles will I be playing five years from now . . . ten . . .and so forth? Is there a role that I would

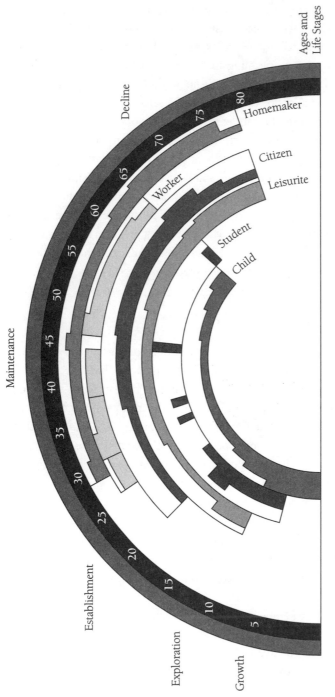

Ages and
Life Stages

Decline

Maintenance

Establishment

Exploration

Growth

Homemaker

Citizen

Leisurite

Worker

Student

Child

5 10 15 20 25 30 35 40 45 50 55 60 65 70 75 80

FIGURE 8   The Life Career Rainbow: Six Life Roles in Schematic Space

Note: From "Life Career Rainbow" by Donald E. Super, in the *Journal of Vocational Behavior*, 1980, Orlando, FL: Academic Press. Copyright 1980 by Academic Press. Reprinted with permission.

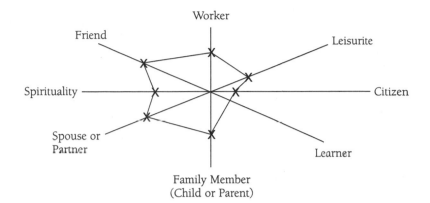

FIGURE 9   Kemp's Variation of Life Career Rainbow

Note: Reprinted with permission of Linda K. Kemp.

like to change? What do I need to do to change my role? Am I mixing up the theaters in which my roles are played and thereby confusing my life? Am I bringing my work role home and disrupting my family? Am I neglecting to play the role of student? Do I need to learn how to parent?

Linda K. Kemp, a career development specialist and a director of management training and development for the United States Postal Service, developed an interesting assessment tool based on Super's Rainbow. She took six roles from the rainbow, added two more, and placed them as equidistant vectors radiating from a central point, shown in Figure 9. The two added roles are *friend* and *spirituality*. Spirituality is called a role because it may include, but is not limited to, being a parishioner, congregant, or church member. Persons are asked to place a mark on each of the eight vectors indicating the present amount of waking time they spend in each role. They are then told to connect the marks so that the diagram may look like the one in Figure 9. It assumes the configuration of whatever the person working with it sees as his or her life space.

The next question to be asked is whether the configuration looks like a desirable one. If not, what would be a desirable one? The participant is asked to draw the desirable configuration. This configuration can be completed on the same design as the other using either dotted lines or a color to distinguish the two chartings. Now the question is how to get to the desired position. What needs to be given up, and what needs to be

Assign each force an intensity rating equal to the strength of that factor as a restraining or contributing force. Place an intensity rating in each circle. (1 = not much; 6 = very much)

Restraining Forces
(keep you from reaching your goal)

Contributing Forces
(help you to reach your goal)

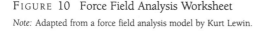

Goal

Date goal is to
be achieved

FIGURE 10   Force Field Analysis Worksheet

Note: Adapted from a force field analysis model by Kurt Lewin.

acquired to arrive at where one wants to be? A force field analysis might be useful in resolving the dilemma, where restraining forces and contributing forces are analyzed in relation to one's goal, as seen in Figure 10.

Instead of using goal setting, Miller-Tiedeman (1989) talks about using one's career compass (experience, intelligence, and intuition) to determine one's course, and then of setting one's intentions to get to the place perceived to be desirable or valuable. Miller-Tiedeman's theory, Lifecareer, talks about life as the big career and about life-as-career in terms of how the career journey is lived. Principles of the new physics, including uncertainty and complementary along with biological principles related to self-organizing systems, constitute the underpinnings of this theory. Self-conceiving and responsibility, cooperation with life, and trust are important elements. Lifecareer theory tells one that believing is seeing and that "it all depends" is the answer to many questions.

CONCLUSION

This chapter has been an attempt to link assessment with the growing field of spirituality and career development. The chapter ends where it began by saying that what we see depends on how we look at things and/or who is doing the looking. The theories presented in this chapter are by no means all-inclusive. Each expresses a point of vision—a way of looking at things and a way of understanding them. The assessment exercises based on theory are intended to do the same. They represent a way, not all ways, of looking at self in the world: a way that can be related to work and to life lived as career.

There are powerful metaphors that can be used to describe and assess one's career journey. It can be compared to the journey of the Israelites through the desert with all of the barrenness and the hunger that the people experienced. The metaphors within that metaphor, such as the building of the golden calf and the receiving of manna, can be used to illustrate personal experiences.

St. Paul's ocean voyages, with his frequent experience of being shipwrecked, is another interesting metaphor. We too experience seas of discontent and winds of change. In the end, we can return to the original metaphor for this chapter, a story the author first learned in childhood, the metaphor of the rabbi of Nemirov, in the hope that we too, through our life's work, can ascend to our own heaven—or perhaps higher.

NOTE

1. The original story by I. L. Peretz (1851–1915) was written in Yiddish. An English translation of "If Not Higher" appears in a book entitled *Selected Stories* edited by Irving Howe and

Eliezer Greenberg, Schocken Books, 1974. "If Not Higher" can also be found in *Stories and Pictures by Isaac Loeb Peretz* (1947), translated from the Yiddish by Helena Frank, Philadelphia, The Jewish Publication Society of America. The story told here is an adaptation, as the author remembers it, of the Peretz story, told to her in her youth by a storyteller. It approximates the original but does not catch the nuances.

REFERENCES

Adler, A. (1956). *The individual psychology of Alfred Adler: A systematic presentation in selection from his writings* (H. L. Ansbacher & R. R. Ansbacher, Eds.). New York: Basic Books.

Adler, A. (1979). *Superiority and social interest: A collection of later writings* (3rd ed.) (H. L. Ansbacher & R. R. Ansbacher, Eds.). New York: Norton.

Bolles, R. N. (1997). *The 1997 What Color Is Your Parachute?* Berkeley, CA: Ten Speed Press.

Fox, M. (1995). *The reinvention of work* (paperback ed.). San Francisco: Harper San Francisco.

Frankle, V. E. (1963). *Man's search for meaning* (rev. ed.). Boston: Beacon Press.

Holland, J. L. (1973). *Making vocational choices: A theory of careers.* Englewood Cliffs, NJ: Prentice Hall.

Holland, J. L. (1985). *Making vocational choices: A theory of vocational personalities and work environments* (2nd ed.). Englewood Cliffs, NJ: Prentice Hall.

Holland, J. L. (1989). *The occupation finder for use with the Self-Directed Search.*™ Odessa, FL: Psychological Assessment Resources.

Holland, J. L. (1990). *Self-Directed Search assessment booklet* (Form R). Odessa, FL: Psychological Assessment Resources.

Holland, J. L., Powell, A., & Fritzsche, B. A. (1994). *The Self-Directed Search professional user's guide.* Odessa, FL: Psychological Assessment Resources.

Jung, C. G. (1933). *Modern man in search of a soul* (W. S. Dell & C. F. Baynes, Trans.). New York: Harcourt Brace & World. (Original work published in 1931.)

Merriam-Webster's Collegiate Dictionary (10th ed.). (1993). Springfield, MA: Merriam-Webster.

Miller-Tiedeman, A. (1989). *How NOT to make it . . . and succeed: The truth about your lifecareer.* Vista, CA: Lifecareer® Foundation.

Peretz, I. L. (1974). *Selected stories* (I. Howe & E. Greenberg, Eds.). New York: Schocken Books.

Rayburn, C., & Richmond, L. J. (1966). Inventory of spirituality. Unpublished assessment instrument, Loyola College.

Schein, E. H. (1990). *Career anchors: Discovering your real values.* San Diego: Pfeiffer.

Super, D. E. (1984). Career and life development. In D. Brown & L. Brooks (Eds.), *Career choice and development: Applying contemporary approaches to practice.* San Francisco: Jossey-Bass.

Super, D. E. (1980). Life Career Rainbow. *Journal of Vocational Behavior, 16,* 282–298. Orlando, FL: Academic Press.

Sweeney, T. J., & Witmer, J. M. (1991). Beyond social interest: Striving toward wholeness. *Industrial Psychology, 47* (4), 527–540.

U.S. Department of Labor (1991). *Dictionary of occupational titles* (4th ed.- rev.). Washington, DC: U.S. Government Printing Office.

Wicks, R. J. (1995). *Seeds of sensitivity.* Notre Dame, IN: Ave Maria Press.

Witmer, J. M., & Sweeney, T. J. (1992). A holistic model of wellness and prevention over the life span. *The Journal of Counseling and Development, 71,* 140–148.

CHAPTER ELEVEN

Inspiriting the Workplace

Developing a Values-Based Management System

Samuel M. Natale
College of St. Scholastica

Joanne C. Neher
College of St. Scholastica

THE TERM *value-based management* is redundant because all human actions are based upon values. The question that needs to be addressed is, what value, and why? In the context of this chapter, "value" is equated with "ethic." It is important to remember that an ethical person is viewed as always doing the right thing in his or her personal as well as professional life. This is directly related to the type of work a person chooses, as well as his or her feeling of success, fulfillment, frustration, and understanding of failure versus achievement. What constitutes work as "activity" or "value" is clearly both social and personal in nature, with occupation meaning not only what one does but also who one is. The meaning of work, then, is conceived from a highly individualized "network of direct and indirect influences or associations" (Hall, 1986, p. 169), resulting in an inherent subjectivity to the concept. In short, work is what we define it to be.

Some years ago, the authors observed a scenario involving a young couple in their thirties at a Sunday afternoon cocktail party with a guest list of fifty people carefully chosen from the high ranks of the business and political world. The husband, a college professor with a doctorate in economics, was appointed by then mayor of New York City, Abraham Beam, to serve on the Commission on Temporary Finance—the mayor's "blue ribbon" group. Each guest was graciously introduced first by title and then by name. The professor's wife stood by as her husband was introduced repeatedly around the room as "Dr. X., who is on the mayor's commission," and we observed that a slight nod went in the direction of the woman, "and his wife." Her own name and the fact that she was "working" as a housewife and mother of her three small children was never mentioned. Well into the festivities of the afternoon, she stood in the company of four people whose positions were honored. Another guest, an older *grande dame,* made her way over to the esteemed group for introductions. She turned to the professor's wife, saying, "I've been talking to your husband about the mayor's commission. I didn't quite understand from him, however, just what it is that you do." The professor's wife looked this *grande dame* directly in the eye, sipped a bit of champagne, and replied without flinching, "Laundry." The older woman did not respond; however, the look of bemused condescension on her face spoke volumes. This interaction demonstrates yet another lesson regarding the values and individual definitions of *work* and *workplace.*

THE PROTESTANT WORK ETHIC.

The Protestant Work Ethic (PWE), as encapsulated by Weber in 1904, glorified work as "a way by which [humanity] could prove [itself]" and as a "means to serve God" (Weber, 1946, p. 96). The PWE understands work as something other than a punishment. The PWE excludes no one from participating in work—thereby furthering each person's ultimate role and contribution of efforts through that work to bring about the Kingdom of God.

As Leech (1977) points out, recent secularization prevents a belief in God from acting as a basis for the meaning of work. This is the result of "a collapse of the Christian basis of culture" (p. 169). Similarly Cherrington (1980) indicates that since the ecumenical movement of the early 1950s, there have been very few articles published in the mainstream press that attempt to "justify diligence and hard work as a commandment of God" (p. 2). As Inks states today, "The PWE represents only one facet of the work values construct" (1992, p. 7). Articles such as this point toward the advent of a culture in which the "God of conventional Western theism" no longer acts as the primary justification for the concept of work. *The Economist* points out that there is a growing tendency among workers to draw a clear line between their work lives and their private lives ("*The Lure of Leisure,*" 1992). The significance of this trend cannot be underestimated.

At a recent family celebration, a group of young and very successful salespeople were talking about the sudden death of a fellow salesperson— a thirty-eight-year-old father of five children, the victim of a massive heart attack. After their contemporary's death had been outlined to them, there was a momentary pause, and one of the members of the group asked quite casually, "Has anyone heard who is getting his territory?" This callous and uncaring attitude is all too pervasive in our society today.

There are far too many of these experiences in our desensitized, efficiency-oriented workplaces. The individual scenarios may change, but the core remains the same. We strive for success; we have inherited the PWE of duty, responsibility, and efficiency. We are taught to work hard, to have far-reaching plans, to have goals well ordered and tasks clearly defined. We are to be cooperative; we follow the rules by transcending self-interest as we become part of the large company or institution.

We are a far cry from the concept of work mentioned earlier: work perceived as the central focus and influence of life, which combines humanity and God in bringing to us the Kingdom of God. At that level, workers performed whatever work there was to be done as a call to greatness, fulfilling the potential in an aura of freedom. Duty was a "holy undertaking," and business was a service to humanity. Without attaching success or failure to the outcome, a person focused on the pride of a job well done for its own sake. To the work alone, then, did the person have the right, with God deciding the fruits of the labor.

THE WORK ETHIC OF TODAY

The world today does not value the honor in work as it did in the Middle Ages. Even at the height of "success," passion in the workplace has been replaced by the ever-present feelings of insecurity at a time of mergers and downsizing. Fear and aggression have replaced joy, honor, and pride, resulting in an inescapable and universal malaise. We have compromised and damaged ourselves to the core of our souls, and our spirits need to heal. At the heart of our shared human condition, our potential yearns to be set free, but we are stifled and blocked, left gasping and out of breath. Where are we going that we do not have time for enjoyment? Or as Wordsworth said, "The world is too much with us; late and soon, getting and spending, we lay waste our powers; little we see in Nature that is ours, we have given our hearts away, a sordid boon!" (Wordsworth, 1888, p. 1806)

This lack of spirit in the workplace is a reflection of the attitudes of the men and women who participate in its process. It can be traced to the fears, warped aspirations, maimed self-images, and general self-centeredness of human beings. The all-pervasive influence of material consumption has led generations of people into choices that place objects above people, profit above human costs, and present gratification over concern for future generations. Changes must be made so that institutions can reshape their self-understanding while transforming their corporate identities. Structures that have by definition acquired a sacred permanency are the nature of a corporation. Tampering with these structures is to alter the way things are "supposed to be." In effect, such tampering means to literally revolutionize our lives and our work ethic to create a new value-based system that allows the emergence of spirit and soul. What is needed here is a transformation from ego to spirit.

We need to redefine the good life as it is equated with purchasing power. The dream of the home in the suburbs as fulfillment and success brings with it the fears of losing all that we have worked so hard to attain. We rightly have a sense of personal pride and accomplishment; however, this must be coupled with a real sense of connectedness to the world at large. In "making it," we must begin an exploration of the questions of integrity, human consequences, rootlessness, and salvation. How misguided is our identification of happiness, and how blind is our pursuit?

SATISFACTION IN WORK

If, as the modern secular world would have it, we can no longer rely on the existence of God as the source from which meanings of work have their genesis, can a sense of *vocatio* still exist? Is there more to work than just making a living or a profit from our daily striving? Is it plausible to suggest that we work simply as a means of basic survival? After all, Braude argues, "because work . . . has become secular . . . it has been shorn of the religious overlay that presumably provided a rational basis for the concept" (1975, p. 8). What can become a rational basis for work beyond the obvious notion that work is a means to feed and shelter ourselves and our families?

Generally speaking, researchers have designated four major reasons for which people work: (1) The work is intrinsically satisfying; (2) the work is a means of survival; (3) the work provides a level of "social connectedness" to the larger community. These first three reasons operate on a continuum and are not limiting. An individual may view his or her work according to any combination of these reasons. Lastly and most importantly, (4) work can also be an intrinsically important activity that contributes to the worker's positive self-perception. Researchers such as Loscocco, Vroom, and Sekaran argue the necessity of viewing work in these terms because work contributes "strongly to self-definition and self-evaluation" (Loscocco, 1985, p. 10). Essentially, the worker's identity merges *with the work* and results in the work becoming a central factor in self-understanding. In order for this positive self-perception to occur, specific characteristics must be present. One is that the work provide the worker with "autonomy control" or an amount of personal control that the worker has in regard to the pace of the work and the level of involved decision making.

If autonomy and safety are present, the worker can express him- or herself positively within the work. Loscocco (1985) theorizes that along with autonomy there must be intrinsic rewards as well; that is, the existence of challenge, meaning, and variety—which "will have a strong positive impact on work commitment" (p. 65). Loscocco points to various studies that conclude that if the work is performed for intrinsic pleasures that spring from a variety of engaging tasks, then a degree of commitment to that work is generated.

Researchers theorize that many workers view their work as a means of obtaining "social connectedness." Feelings of depersonalization and alienation indicate that work must serve as a center of social growth. These social systems "exist as a result of human proclivities, of all the unwritten contracts that grow up between a company and its employees" (Zaleznik, 1989, p. 58). This social dimension of work, as an extrinsic reward, inhibits people from viewing work "as something which only provides economic rewards" (Loscocco, 1985, p. 68).

Social interaction and approval are then necessary but not sufficient conditions for the possibility of satisfaction: "Employees who perform highly fragmented tasks are not more likely to look for work for self-expression simply because of satisfying relationships" (Loscocco, p. 68). If the work itself does not provide any significant level of fulfillment or a means by which the worker can express him- or herself, the social dimension of that work will not provide that self-fulfillment. Here work means the paycheck; that is, food, shelter, and clothing. It is evident today that this attitude toward work as a wholly unfulfilling yet necessary action is a prevalent and commonly held conception (Hollencamp, 1985).

In *Converting 9 to 5,* Haughey (1990) comments on the effect of anonymity and the impossibility of extracting any substantial meaning from work unless personal involvement to work and the workplace is achieved. He argues that workers are currently experiencing a severe detachment from today's workplace. To alleviate this, Haughey proposes a nationwide "universal stock ownership" plan in which the 94 percent of the population who do not have investments in the stock market would receive government loans to purchase such stock. Such a program will provide workers with the fundamental connection to the work environment, a connection that Haughey believes is largely absent from our culture.

The idea of work has a variety of meanings, dependent upon particular characteristics of work as well as individual perceptions of work. Work that contains a higher level of autonomy is more likely to be an enjoyable activity, which would create an environment for more self-expression. Conversely, work that controls the worker is more likely to be viewed as an unfortunate but necessary obligation of existence. There is also the view that work fulfills social need, providing the worker with a "social connection" to the larger community. Within these parameters, meaning and work are in tension with each other in such a way that the experience of one anticipates the other (Hall, 1986).

VALUES REDISCOVERED

A renewal of vitality in our values, attitudes, needs, and expectations cannot be achieved simply by bringing in consultants. Nor can we achieve success by bringing back the old values or religious beliefs. In fact, Ronco and Peattie (1990) include a European values study—an international report prepared by a number of scholars and social scientists—which affirms that secularism is flourishing in western Europe. The study reports that Europeans view religion as less significant to their lives than family, friends, work, and leisure activity. The impact of religion declined most sharply in Scandinavia and northwest Europe, where less than half the population views religion as very important. Fewer than half of all Belgians, Britons, Dutch, French, Germans, and Scandinavians expressed confidence in their churches. Are Western societies becoming less religious, or are their practices changing?

Encouraging Education

It is not our intention to list concerns without redress. In fact, it is encouraging to understand that the solution (deliverance) must come from an educational approach to the problem, an approach that calls together affective, behavioral, and cognitive components in nations, corporations, and individuals to establish a new foundation to search for meaning. Many people have forgotten the ideals of the work ethic—thrift, industry, diligence, and perseverance. Restoration of the work ethic requires teaching it to children in the home as well as to the culture at large. Six values need to be emphasized: (1) value of the worker; (2) value of leaders; (3) value of responsibility and pursuit of excellence; (4) value of training; (5) value of economic and humane profit; and (6) value of leadership that enables others to meet goals (Colson & Eckerd, 1992).

Educationally, these problems are considerable. What we're speaking of is the belief that all values are subjective functions of the individual rather than principles rooted in the wisdom of the ages. Children are taught to let their conscience be their guides. However, children do not have the experience to decide what their consciences should hold dear. This surrenders to the notion that one cannot hope for any kind of unified moral vision, a concept that is often upheld as "pluralism" or "diversity." Yet pluralism and diversity suggest valuing differences only. They do not suggest a lack of parameters that circumscribe morally educated behavior (Neff, 1992).

The president of the Association for Humanistic Psychology, in addressing the thirtieth annual conference (O'Hara, 1992), writes that the values that lie at the core of the humanistic psychology movement have a great deal to offer a pluralistic culture. In the early days of the movement, the emphasis was on self-realization through inner work. It is now clear that people must reconnect and make a commitment to each other, to their communities, and to the Earth they share.

Seeking Balance

This goal of connection and commitment is not easily achieved. We must name the demon, ferret it out of our psyche, and then make a choice. The goal will be determined by our choices, and the reward will be growth and a revitalization of our personal and collective concept of work. What we need most of all is a balance, and there are many "escape routes" that we can take to heighten the imbalance.

Identity One way of avoiding a heightened awareness of our needs and vulnerability is by ignoring our need for interdependence by asserting our own independence and strength. Many people throw themselves into work, becoming overextended to the exclusion of forming relationships. Individual personality becomes merged with corporate identity, a kind of belligerent independence and manipulation under the guise of excellence and importance. How often are people introduced at social gatherings by a job title, lending prestige to both the party being introduced and the person making the introduction? Idolatry knows no boundaries; it infiltrates and engulfs our personal lives and contaminates the very air we breathe.

Ego Does the meaning of a job lie in the joy and challenge of the work, or only in the money it pays? Many jobs that truly help others are looked down upon and/or passed over because they do not pay large salaries. Our value lies in what you do rather than who you are and what you stand for. We live in blue collar or white collar neighborhoods; we seek upwardly mobile acquaintances; we marry the corporate wife or husband. People want to network rather than develop real human bonds; they want to fill their address books with names and phone numbers of the important contacts they can make, enabling them to reap an even more luscious harvest. Inspiriting the workplace has to begin here. Do we live our lives according to the ego rather than the spirit? It is difficult when we focus on the "rewards" to remember that we are called upon to do an honest day's work for an honest day's wage.

Weakness How often is energy wasted on aggression when it can be better used for the journey within? How many people hide behind their own competence and a veneer of concern for others instead of focusing on their own longings and limitations? We need to learn to think in a way that is not exclusive to intelligence, capability, or professional success. We must incorporate an assessment of our strong and weak points as well as our wants and needs.

Hedonism Another escape route is to a kind of hedonism, which is acted out in "liquid lunches" and "let it all hang out" Christmas parties when alcohol loosens the tongue. We sometimes misuse our senses of touching, tasting, seeing, smelling, and hearing to turn off our awareness of our own inner emptiness. People long for tenderness and affirmation—and experience a desire to pour out their very souls—to let their spirits soar. But at the core, there is an emptiness that people feel; they know that there is something missing, and it will not go away by denying its existence.

Responsibility Entering a fantasy world of overactive imagination is yet another barrier; however, we must understand that we are responsible for our own actions. We can be overly defensive rather than take responsibility and correct our errors. Many lash out by putting up a defense against the company or society as a whole. At times, it is difficult being responsible for one's own actions. We can look at a situation through logic and acceptance of the facts and then harness the power within us to change.

Anger Unresolved anger is another "escape route." It leads to further hurt, not only to ourselves but to others as well. We sometimes have medical problems that are work related in origin, accompanied by real pain and real physical damage. Medical experts agree that anger and emotional wounds can manifest in medical illnesses and physical accidents. The inner problem becomes visible in our outer physical self (i.e., asthma attacks, a physical feeling of being "choked," literally suffocated by the anger that we have been trying to stifle).

Effecting Change

Clarification and confrontation are the only ways to effect real change. Just "knowing" that we have hope (or no hope) for a raise or a better job is not enough. We have to assess what our accomplishments are and what the requirements would be for a new role. We must objectify ourselves to see both strengths and weaknesses so we can build on one and counteract the other, respectively. No step in a positive direction can be taken unless we see ourselves as we really are.

What is called for on the corporate communal level and on a personal level is a radical empowerment to enact change: a call for competency, cooperation, control, communication, and caring within the workplace. We are engaged in "business" that is much more than business, and "profit" that must be measured in more than productivity, dollars, and power. We are calling for a radical change on the level of human spirit, where choices and actions are based on mutual responsibility, accountability, honor, and pride, replacing helplessness, fear, mistrust, and passive acceptance of "the way things are." We are asking the business industry and workers to shape events, rather than be shaped by them. Workers need to be totally present—mind, body, spirit, and soul—to enkindle a renewed reverence for human ability and creativity.

SPIRITUALITY IN THE WORKPLACE

First of all, it is necessary to see that corporate culture and a true spirituality in the workplace can coexist. They balance one another; they are complementary and inclusive. Table 3 shows how this balance works.

The effort to infuse the corporate culture with spirituality must be approached on several levels. As stated earlier, an educational approach to achieving new meaning in the workplace, to infusing spirituality, must include affective, behavioral, and cognitive components that address the meaning of spirituality on the national, corporate, and individual levels. Only by a systems approach—reconnecting the components of the corporate environment with the personal systems of the worker—can there be a restoration of the work ethic, where people believe in the value of work, where work means more than a paycheck. The question becomes one of "how to" rather than "should we?" However, even agreeing on this question can be difficult. It must be approached on three levels: national, corporate, and individual. Of course, there are sublevels within each of these systems, but methods of infusion into these sublevels become the unique focus of each major component of the system. The emphasis here is on the big

TABLE 3   Corporate Culture and Spirituality

Corporate Culture	Spirituality
External authority/rules	Internal authority
Cultural and ethnic	Personal and individualistic
Organizational code	Experiential
Hierarchical structure	Inner integrity/interiority
Institutional	Prophetic
Form	Content
Accountability (corporate)	Discernment of abilities
Thinking	Feeling

Note: From *The Difference Between Religion and Spirituality,* by P. McCall, 1992, New York: House of Peace. Adapted with permission.

picture, on the overriding structures affecting each person. Specific methods for this infusion are needed. Although these may vary among management systems, there are some general suggestions for how to approach this reintegration. Agreement must be reached that values have utility within management systems. The question then becomes one of how to best address these values.

Defining Mission

The approach taken here is that a systems method of infusion is necessary to effect change. Nations have the equivalent of mission statements in their constitutions or other founding documents. Corporations usually have something equivalent to a mission statement, which provides an overview of the values upheld by management. The missions articulated by nations and corporations are guiding principles used to shape these systems. How much these statements are used varies with the systems, from one end of the continuum where all decisions are mission statement based to the other end where the statement is a nice document to have but where it is also not a guiding force used in the everyday operations of the system. Individuals rarely have a formal mission statement as such. However, they do have guiding principles by which they measure their behavior. These principles come from personal belief systems and may be formulated from religious beliefs, from family systems, from private development of the self, or from a combination of these factors. The alienation of the individual from the workplace and from production comes from a separation of these individual belief systems from the mission statements of nations and corporations. The question then becomes one of how to reconnect these systems, these values, in such a way that the employee feels a sense of connectedness with the job and where the employee receives intrinsic reward for work produced.

Turning Principles into Action

One of the difficulties in attempting this reconstruction is in recognizing that there is distance between these levels of systems. Most people would say that they uphold the values stated in their country's founding documents. These same people would likely say that they agree with the missions of their employing systems. The loftiness of these statements may then be the problem. Guiding principles are usually broad, allowing for a wide diversity in interpretation. Translating these principles into everyday interactions is the function of the three levels of systems: national, corporate, and individual. These translations are matters of choice: Which values will be addressed? How much emphasis will each value receive? Which values will be sacrificed for expediency or profit or situation? Can there even be agreement on the values? Does their very nonspecificity cause them to be nice ideas that are shelved for the sake of efficiency? Does an employee even need to be concerned with the values of the system within which work is done, or does the employee only need to be concerned about "the job"? This chapter provides a method of reinfusion of values into management. The search for meaning is becoming more evident as the alienation of the worker from the workplace is increasing. This search for meaning can be the grounding concept around which spirituality can be reintroduced.

We propose that there can be a reinfusion of spirit, that there can be a reduction of alienation from the workplace if there is a redirection of effort to focus on those belief systems in a way that coalesces into a commitment to uphold whatever those values are. From a national perspective, this may mean more focus on those founding documents mentioned earlier. How can these statements about how government should work be used to infuse spirit into management systems? Managers and employees should be given the opportunity to articulate how they see the content of these documents fitting into the work environment. There should be clear, specific examples of how a government's values are translated into the corporate system. The focus should be on the management system as the core of a larger corporate system. Management should be guided to see the utility of concrete, measurable objectives based on the corporation's stated mission and goals. The refocusing of mindset can be done through strategies designed for a reinfusion of spirit. Proposals for doing this are as follows:

1. Attention to the founding documents of the governmental system should be articulated in relation to the personnel within the corporate system.
2. There should be an application of values presented in the founding documents to the mission of the corporate structure and to management procedures.
3. Constant clarification of the translation of values into policies and procedures should be evident in the workplace.
4. Personnel at all levels of the system should be involved in the formulation of value statements, policies, and procedures.
5. Within the educational system, modeling of vertical involvement of individuals can be valuable.
6. Confrontation within the system, whether corporate, educational, or familial, should focus on maintaining articulated values.

IMPLICATIONS FOR VALUE-BASED MANAGEMENT PROCEDURES

As Flynn (1995, p. 32) states, "Well-communicated guidelines help set the parameters for employees." We propose that a formalized procedure for orientation, ongoing discussion, clarification, and confrontation can facilitate the reinfusion of spirit into the corporate structure. There must be a clearly explicated policy in place, with procedures, understood by all levels of the corporation, that are followed consistently. Specific strategies for application of this policy are discussed as follows.

Founding Documents

Infusion of the content of governmental documents can be designed within the orientation meetings of new employees. A clear, specific discussion about the meaning of government rules, regulations, and philosophy as these pertain to the specific internal and external workings of the corporation can be the beginning of building a value-based system. This discussion can be done within the context of how new regulations affect the corporate structure. Snow and Bloom (1996) recommend using a combination of lecture and case study to incorporate content about values and ethics into the education of managers, as well as into the MBA classroom. In testing this method, they have found that lectures can provide an overview of whatever policy must be applied to specific situations, but managers are much more capable of translating values into practice when they are involved in discussions about issues that directly relate to their levels of involvement in the corporation. Within the broader context of social responsibility, practice in articulation of management issues and strategies can enhance the corporate environment and can extend into the community.

Corporate Mission Statements

Once management has a grasp on how the corporate structure shapes and is shaped by government-based values, more attention can be paid to the development and articulation of mission statements. These statements must not be merely nice overgeneralizations of the purpose of the corporation. Mission statements should be guiding principles applied daily in the structure and functions of the work environment. Decisions should be based on this statement and articulated in terms of the mission. There should be a clear, specific linkage between the idealism of the mission and the everyday workings of the system.

This can only come through clarification and confrontation, through efforts to involve the components of the system; that is, the employees at all levels, in a constant focus on this link. This can be done, again, through workshops that are a regular part of the structure of management. Consistent review of mission as it affects daily decision making is built into the agenda. As Flynn (1995) states, "A good ethics program provides both verbal and written reinforcement" (p. 34). Infusion of values should be in oral form and in print, distributed to managers and employees. Availability of what ethics mean, of how values are part of the everyday work process, greatly enhances productivity and morale.

Translation of Values into Policies and Procedures

Management and employees should be expected to read the mission statements that guide their corporations. Corporate leadership must be very clear about the necessity for decision making based on the mission. Any policy or procedure within the corporate structure should be formulated in light of the mission of that system. Regular review is a necessary component of translation, at least every three months, or whenever new environmental issues will affect the corporation, or at whatever "natural" review points exist in the system. This could be as simple as completing goals and objectives for each sector of the system, which are clearly linked to the mission, printed, and distributed. It could be as time consuming as weekly team meetings where there is consistent reevaluation of the mission, goals and objectives, and policies of the system. Flynn (1995) recommends that handouts, booklets, and a regular system of information distribution become part of the corporate structure, that all levels of the system know the linkages, know where to access information, and know how to proceed when there is tension between stated value-based policies and actual observed behaviors. Thus clarification and articulation of policies are dynamic and span all levels of the corporation.

Involving All Levels of the System

Administration, management, and employees have an ongoing vested interest in the structure and function of the system, based on a clearly specified value base. Once this base is in place, it becomes a guiding force for everyday decision making. Employees at all levels have a framework within which decisions can be made, based on the documents and discussions about values that have taken place. This takes high-level corporate commitment. It also takes alteration of the traditional hierarchical management system. Within training sessions, workshops, and regular planning sessions, multilevel involvement is necessary. When management uses values in developing working structures, this demonstrates model behavior for employees. As more power is delegated to online staff, there is a stronger need for practicing decision making through case study scenarios similar to those faced by the system. Where employees have direct experience in applying values to daily tasks, production rises and morale improves. This happens simply because personnel have the chance to practice "what if" questions, to test their own decision making skills, and to receive support from the corporate structure in this process.

Education Strategies

To reinfuse spirit into management, people need to bring an understanding of how to do this to the job. This can be done by a recommitment to values within components of the education system. School is a training ground for work, for the work ethic, for development of personal and professional values. Although some would argue that children should not be included in the articulation of values and policies in their education, Iannone (1989) would disagree. The education system is where people begin to formulate the values they will use in group situations as adults. This includes those values carried into employment. The commitment that is needed from management can also be obtained from educational administrators. Parents, teachers, administrators, and students can be involved in translating values into educational systems. This is more than the expectation that parents become involved in PTA systems. Just as corporate structures should articulate missions, goals, and objectives in light of values, this same format can be used in education. Ongoing discussions, scheduled when all levels of the education system can be present, can increase the understanding of values and of how these values are carried out in the classroom. Allowing children access to this process, on a level at which they can contribute, begins to instill in them the understanding that input is valuable, that there is a link between them and the systems within which they function. By modeling a systems approach, where a variety of perspectives is honored, empowerment for all components of the system can be improved.

This method can be applied to education from primary grades through graduate coursework. The case scenario format can be extremely effective in aiding those in the education system in development of a value-based perspective. Again, participants can be encouraged to test their own styles, to question and formulate values that will help them address questions similar to those faced within the everyday workings of the education system. Values and ethics courses, or lessons within broader curricula, should be an important part of education, not left to elective courses in college liberal arts studies. (One of the authors of this chapter, in dealing with a student who once cheated on an exam, was treated to the explanation that ethics did not matter in this student's life; he was going into sports management! There is something wrong when a student has this perspective.) Ongoing, consistent clarification of the purpose of ethics in personal and professional tasks should be practiced. Internalization of the importance of ethics, as well as strategies for employing ethics in practice, should be goals of the education system at all levels. Specific, measurable educational objectives can be made clear in this system. This proposal does not imply that there is one "right" way to solve ethical dilemmas or that there is one "right" value to be applied. Education should provide the tools necessary to formulate strategies for decision making. Situations vary; people are diverse. Processes can allow for variation in problem solving and diversity of outcomes. Persons within the education system can be given many opportunities to test out their values through role plays, case scenarios, and discussions where diverse perspectives are honored. Attention to real-life problems can foster development of a value base that is useful in corporate structures.

Even if the above strategies are integrated into corporate and educational systems, there will be conflict and differences in how values should be applied. This leads to a discussion about how confrontation can be used in value-based management.

Maintaining a Focus on Articulated Values

The discussion of education strategies assumes that there will be a clearly articulated system of values within corporate, educational, and familial structures. If this is true, then confrontation over the application of values can be minimized. However, there will always be conflict as people bring diverse perspectives to any situation. When confrontation is necessary, it should be done within the framework of value-based decision making. When personnel have had practice in thinking through decisions, they may have less difficulty when decisions and policies must be challenged. Having a structure in place where confrontation is allowed, where there are several options for obtaining assistance in difficult situations, can serve the corporation well. W. Michael Hoffman, executive director of the Center for Business Ethics, recommends that employees have several choices available for clarification on value dilemmas. He recommends the use of open communication among levels of the system, written requests, meetings where the employee is comfortable (possibly where that employee won't be seen talking to the ethics officer), and anonymous requests. He always recommends confidentiality in value discussions. This ensures safety as well as smooths the way for hesitant employees to come forward with concerns. If careful attention has been given to the clear definition of values within the corporate system, confrontation can be reduced. When confrontation is necessary, it must be welcomed and supported. Perhaps there will be dissonance between the belief systems of the employee and that of the company. It then becomes the responsibility of each component to evaluate if this dissonance can be tolerated, or if the "fit" between system and individual is too poor to continue functioning. This then becomes the responsibility of each party to decide on the future of the employee within that system.

CONCLUSION

At Texas Instruments, a checklist of questions is used as a guide for employees when they are making decisions. These questions include the following:

1. Is the action legal?
2. Does it comply with our values?
3. If you do it, will you feel bad?
4. How will it look in the newspaper?
5. If you know it's wrong, don't do it.
6. If you're not sure, ask.
7. Keep asking until you get an answer.

Note: From "Make Employee Ethics Your Business," by G. Flynn, June 1995, *Personnel Journal,* p. 34. Reprinted with permission.

None of the proposals discussed in this chapter assumes that there is one truth, one set of values upon which an entire system can agree. There is room for diversity in these proposals. The process of clarification does not imply agreement on every value, or even on a majority of values. If attention is placed on continual articulation of values, on their meaning in everyday management of a system, there is room for negotiation. Reconnection with the workplace should come when more and more of the spirit of individuals and the spirit of management can be understood and applied to the goals and objectives of the system; that is, when mission statements are infused into the personal spirit of employees.

REFERENCES

Braude, L. (1975). *Work and workers.* New York: Praeger.

Cherrington, D. J. (1980). *The work ethic.* New York: Amacom.

Colson, C. W., & Eckerd, J. M. (1992). *Christianity Today, 36,* 34–7. F

Flynn, G. (1995, June). Make employee ethics your business. *Personnel Journal,* 30–41.

Hall, R. H. (1986). *Dimensions of work.* Beverly Hills: Sage.

Haughey, J. C. (1990). *Converting 9 to 5.* New York: Crossroads.

Hollencamp, P. K. (1985). *What is the experience of the meaning of work.* Doctoral dissertation, cc. Hollencamp, P. K.

Iannone, A. P. (1989). *Contemporary moral controversies in business.* New York: Oxford University Press.

Inks, L. W. (1992). *An interactionist perspective on work value change.* Doctoral dissertation, cc. Inks, L. W.

Inks, L. W. The Lure of Leisure. (1992, May 2). *The Economist.*

Leech, K. (1977). *Soul friend.* London: Sheldon Press.

The lure of leisure. (1992, May 2). *The Economist.*

Loscocco, K. A. (1985). *The meaning of work: An examination of the determinants of work commitment and work orientation among manufacturing employees.* Doctoral dissertation, cc. Loscocco, K. A.

McCall, P. (1992). *The difference between religion and spirituality.* New York: House of Peace.

Neff, D. (1992, August 17). American Babel. *Christianity Today, 36,* 18–19.

O'Hara, M. (1992, August 1). If not now, when? *Vital Speeches of the Day, 59,* 41–45.

Ronco, W., & Peattie, L. (1990). Making work: Secularism's persistence (European values study). *The Christian Century, 108,* 962.

Snow, R. M., & Bloom, A. J. (1996). A survey-based pedagogical approach to ethics in the workplace. *Journal of Applied Behavioral Science, 32*(1), 89–100.

Weber, M. (1946). *From Max Weber: Essays in sociology* (H. H. Gerth & C. Wright Mills, Trans.). New York: Oxford University Press.

Wordsworth, W. (1888). The world is too much with us. In *The Complete Works of William Wordsworth.* London: Macmillan.

Zaleznik, A. (1989). *The managerial mystique.* New York: HarperCollins.

Epilogue

Lee J. Richmond
Loyola College

IS THERE A meaningful link between spirituality and career development? To what extent are the two different, and to what extent are they the same? Phrased another way, is what one does in the world separate from who one is?

Existentialists claim that the human being and the world in which he or she acts form a basic unity. When existentialists speak of being-in-the-world, hyphens are used between the words to accentuate the oneness of subject and object. Creation and co-creators, we humans define our world as we traverse it. Perhaps in doing so, we are our work.

Murphy (1996) suggests a more obscure meaning for spirituality than the common dictionary definition. The common meaning relates to structured religion as it exists outside of the individual. The obscure relates to the root of the word *spirituality—spiritus,* which means *to animate.* By this definition it is the principle of all of life. If spirituality is the life force, the force that sustains and energizes, and if work is the energy spent in creation, whether human or divine (as in Genesis where God works six days out of seven to make a world), then spirit and work are one. Fox, then, is correct when he claims that there is only one great work in the universe and we and our work are a part of it: "All energy is one; indeed *energia* is the Greek word for work" (1995, p. 63).

This book has been about work, meaning in work, and connectedness. It has been about *Dasein,* a German word that means *to exist in the world.* There are three modes of the world that characterize human existence in it: *Umwelt, Mitwelt,* and *Eigenwelt.* The *Umwelt* is the environment around us that would exist even without our awareness of it. The *Mitwelt* refers to our interpersonal relationships. The *Eigenwelt* refers to our inner world—our relationship with ourself.

In our particular time in history, there are many alienated people. The alienated person has no sense of unity between self and world. There is a split between self and environment, self and others, self and self, or perhaps all three. By contrast, the healthy person lives simultaneously in all three worlds. The healthy person is connected. The energy of the cosmos is the spirit of the cosmos, and each such person is a spark that is in, and of, the eternal fire.

Battafarano (1996) writes that career development can be looked at as a process of linking people to tasks, through gifts. Just as we are "constantly changing, and being created anew, so are our world's needs in flux, evolving every day" (p. 6). Through our tasks, says Battafarano, "we bring order out of chaos and touch the divine. Our tasks may be menial. We may operate machinery, deliver mail, pick fruit, dispense tickets, sell merchandise, or clean cesspools; nevertheless, through these tasks, we do two things. We bring order to the world and connect to others." (1996, pp. 11–12). However, often people say, "I'm *just a* teacher," or "I'm *just a* letter carrier," or "I'm *just a* mother." If we listen to the spirit, we know that there are no "just a's." To the one who wants to learn, a teacher is a cherished guide. To the person who awaits a letter from a loved one, the letter carrier is a sacred messenger. To the needy child, a mother is no less than protector and wonderful counselor.

This book has been about the quest for meaning in work and the connection between spirit and career. We have explored work and its meaning through the filters of theology, philosophy, psychology, career development theory, contemporary physics, and quantum mechanics. We have examined intentionality, assessment tools, business ethics, and story. All of this we have done for a single purpose—to illustrate the unity between human work and the human spirit.

In 1923, Kahlil Gibran wrote what became a very popular book, *The Prophet*. The book has been reprinted many times. Perhaps there is no better way to end this book than to listen to the often recited but little heard words of Gibran as related to work:

> You work that you might keep pace with the earth and the soul of the earth . . .
> All work is empty save when there is love . . . and when you work with love,

you bind yourself to one another and to God . . .

Work is love made visible.

And if you cannot work with love but only with distaste, it is better that you should leave your work and sit at the gate of the temple and take alms of those who work with joy.

Foe if you take bread with indifference, you take a bitter bread . . . and if you grudge the crushing of the grapes, your grudge distills a poison in the wine.

And if you sing as angels and love not the singing you muffle ears to the voices of the day and of the night. (Gibran, 1951, pp. 25–28)

And what is love? Says Teilhard de Chardin (1969), "It is a sacred reserve of energy, and the very blood stream of spiritual evolution."

REFERENCES

Battafarano, G. (1996). *Essay on spirituality, mental health, and career counseling.* Unpublished paper, Loyola College.

Fox, M. (1995). *The reinvention of work: A new vision of livelihood for our time.* San Francisco: Harper San Francisco.

Gibran, K. (1951). *The prophet.* New York: Knopf.

Murphy, S. D. (1996). *How are spirituality, mental health, and career development linked?* Unpublished paper, Loyola College.

Teilhard de Chardin, P. (1969). *Building the earth and the psychological conditions of human unification.* New York: Avon.

Contributors

Deborah P. Bloch, Ph.D., is associate professor in the Department of Organization and Leadership at the University of San Francisco. She has worked as a consultant in the United States and Australia concentrating on career development, information systems, workforce preparation, and underserved populations. She has authored four books for the general public, including *How to Write a Winning Résumé,* and is the author of and reader on the *Head and Heart to Career Success* audiotapes. Past president of the National Career Development Association and of the Association of Computer-Based Systems for Career Information, she is a member of the editorial board of the *Career Planning and Adult Development Journal* and a recipient of the first Distinguished Service Award of the Association of Computer-Based Systems for Career Information, the Resource Award of the Career Planning and Adult Development Network, and the Merit Award of the National Career Development Association.

Michael Demkovich, O.P., received his doctorate from the Catholic University of Louvain in Belgium and has taught systematic theology and philosophy in St. Louis, Missouri, at the Aquinas Institute. He resides in Albuquerque, New Mexico, where he is founding director of the Dominican Ecclesial Institute (DEI), a new model in collaborative, itinerant teaching, and where he facilitates the Catholic Business Forum. He has published in *Louvain Studies, Listening,* and *Studies in Formative Spirituality*, and teaches part of the year at Blackfriars in Oxford, England.

Beverly E. Eanes, B.S.N., M.Ed., Ph.D., has more than thirty years' experience in the field of family health and has been on the faculty of both Columbia Union College and Georgetown University. She has her own private counseling practice. A member of the American Nurses Association, the American Counseling Association, the American Association of Pastoral Counselors, and the National Board for Certified Hypnotherapists, she is a nationally and Maryland-certified counselor and a clinical specialist in psychiatric and mental health nursing. She is past president of the Maryland Association for Religious and Value Issues in Counseling and the Maryland Association for Counseling and Development. Author of the book *Joy: The Dancing Spirit of Love Surrounding You,* Eanes currently serves as director of clinical education for the MS/CAS programs in pastoral counseling at Loyola College in Baltimore.

Harvey L. Huntley, Jr., Doctor of Ministry, is currently senior pastor of the Lutherans in Mission Parish in Auburn, Indiana. Previously he served on the national staff of the Lutheran Church in America, where he held a position in occupational counseling with the Division for Professional Leadership in Philadelphia. He received his degree from the University of Chicago and an Advanced Certificate of Study in career counseling from Johns Hopkins University.

Anna Miller-Tiedeman, Ph.D., is president of the Lifecareer® Foundation in Vista, California. She received the George E. Hill Distinguished Alumni Award from Ohio University and the Outstanding Research Award given by the American Association of Counseling. She has written the new quantum career theory described in *How NOT to Make It . . . And Succeed: Life on Your Own Terms; Lifecareer®: The Quantum Leap into a Process Theory of Career; Lifecareer®: How It Can Benefit You;* and *Easy Does It: 18 Simple and Convenient Life-Direction Strategies.* She has also written numerous articles and chapters in books.

Samuel M. Natale, Ph.D., is Arend J. Sandbulte Professor of Ethics and Management at the College of St. Scholastica in Duluth, Minnesota. Concurrently he is Visiting Fellow of Kellogg College, University of Oxford, England. The author of more than twenty books and numerous articles in professional journals, he is editor-in-chief of two journals: *The International Journal of Value-Based Management,* and *Cross Cultural Management.* He consults for corporations and businesses in the areas of conflict management, values-based management, ethics, and technology management.

Joanne C. Neher, Ph.D., LISW, is a graduate of the social work program at Tulane University and received her doctorate in social work from Saint Louis University. Her consultant work has focused on the CSWE reaccreditation process for undergraduate social work programs. She taught in the Social Work Department of East Tennessee State University for two years before beginning her doctoral studies. Currently she is on the faculty at the College of St. Scholastica, in Duluth, Minnesota, where she taught social work and was chair of the Sociology/Social Work Department for ten years. She presently serves as editorial and conference assistant to the Endowed Chair of Management and Ethics, is a social work licensure supervisor, and does extensive volunteer work with the Diocese of Duluth. Her areas of expertise include ethical management, human behavior, social welfare policy, and social work history.

Carole A. Rayburn, Ph.D., M. Div., is a clinical, consulting, and research psychologist. A fellow of the American Psychological Association, she is a past president of the APA Division on the Psychology of Religion, the Maryland Psychological Association, and the APA Division on Clinical Psychology's Section on the Clinical Psychology of Women. She has researched and published in the areas of clergy stress, leadership in work and religious settings, work and play, and pastoral counseling.

Lee J. Richmond, Ph.D., is professor of education and coordinator of the school counseling program at Loyola College in Baltimore, Maryland, where she also teaches the career development course for the pastoral counseling program. She is a national certified counselor, a national certified career counselor, a licensed psychologist in the state of Maryland, and a past president of the National Career Development Association and of the American Counseling Association. Her most recent publications are in the area of meaning and values in counseling and career assessment. She has co-authored three assessment instruments related to spirituality, morality, and work and has given presentations and workshops on the topic of spirituality and work for the National Career Development Association, the American Counseling Association, and the American Psychological Association.

Mark L. Savickas, Ph.D., is professor and chair in the Behavioral Sciences Department at the Northeastern Ohio Universities College of Medicine and adjunct professor of counseling and human development at Kent State University. He edits *Career Development Quarterly* and serves on editorial boards for the *Journal of Counseling Psychology, Journal of Vocational Behavior, Journal of Career Assessment*, and *Educational Research Journal*. He coedited (with R. Lent) *Convergence in Career Development Theories* (1994) and (with B. Walsh) *Handbook of Career Counseling Theory and Practice* (1996). In 1994, he received the John L. Holland Award for Outstanding Achievement in Career and Personality Research from the Counseling Psychology Division of the American Psychological Association. In 1996, he received the Eminent Career Award from the National Career Development Association.

Marian Stoltz-Loike, Ph.D., is vice president of Windham International and is the practice leader for the firm's cross-cultural and intercultural programs. Her understanding of how culture influences business concerns has contributed to the success of business leaders in North America, South America, Asia, Europe, and Australia. She is the author of *Dual Career Couples: New Perspectives in Counseling* and articles on issues related to culture, dual-career couple concerns, and women's career development. She is a member of the board of trustees of the National Career Development Association and a member of the American Counseling Association. She received her undergraduate degree from Harvard University and her advanced degrees from New York University.

David V. Tiedeman, Ed.D., former professor of education, Harvard Graduate School of Education, presently serves as vice president of the Lifecareer® Foundation in Vista, California, and faculty mentor in education, Walden University. He formerly served as president of the National Institute for the Advancement of Career Education headquartered at the University of Southern California, where he retired as professor (emeritus) of higher and postsecondary education. Tiedeman authored *Career Development: Designing Our Career Machines* and coauthored *Career Development: Choice and Adjustment; Career Development: Exploration and Commitment;* and *Career Development: Designing Self*. In addition, he has written numerous chapters in books as well as many articles.

Index

Abbey, E., 108
ability, theory-based assessment of, 220, 225–26
absorbedness, *vii–viii*, 187
Action: Essay on a Critique and a Science of Practice (Blondel), 51, 52–54
action
  ethical, checklist for, 254
  as a focus, 111
  and meaning, 192–93
  principles and, 248–49
Adler, A., 4, 5, 11, 23, 216, 218
adolescence, development of meaning during, 33, 39–40, 42
adulthood, development of meaning during, 34–35, 40–41
affirmation
  and calling, 167–68
  and intentionality, 197–98, 204
age
  and the development of meaning, 30–35
  meaning and, *ix*
alienation, 258
alterity, 58
"Among School Children" (Yeats), *xi–xii*
analysis, force field, 232
anger, and values, 245
Appalachia Education Laboratory, 92
approximation, experiential, 76
Aquinas, Thomas, 121
Archway of Career Determinants, 36
Aristotle, 49

assessment
  of social role. *See* Life Career Rainbow
  theory-based, of career development, 215–29
Association for Humanistic Psychology, 243
attitude, and Lifecareer, 67
Augustine, 121
automation, effects of, 50
autonomy, 31–32

Barker, J. A., 121
Bath, Karl, 118–19, 120, 124, 126
Bell's theorem, 202
Benedict, 121
Big Brother, The (Leyden), 33
biography, uses of, 9–17
Blondel, Maurice, 51, 52–54, 55, 57
Bolles, Richard, 192, 224
Bradbury, Ray, 97
Business of Paradigms, The: Discovering the Future (Video) (Barker), 95

California Career Conference, 192
calling
  deafness to, 179–82
  described, 163–64, 175–79
  response to, 172
  work as, 122, 128, 132–33
capitalism, 48–49
Capra, F., on the scientific revolution, 63, 64, 67, 68, 76, 77, 78, 89, 94, 127